DR. SANKHU MAJUMDAR

Current Clinical Strategies

History and Physical Examination

2001-2002 Edition

Paul D. Chan, M.D.
Peter J. Winkle, M.D.

Current Clinical Strategies Publishing
www.ccspublishing.com

Digital Book and Updates

Purchasers of this book can download the digital book and updates at the Current Clinical Strategies Publishing internet site: www.ccspublishing.com

Current Clinical Strategies Publishing Inc
27071 Cabot Road
Laguna Hills, California 92653-7012
Phone: 800-331-8227
Fax: 800-965-9420
E-mail: info@ccspublishing.com
Internet: www.ccspublishing.com

Printed in USA   ISBN 1881528-812

Contents

Medical Documentation

History and Physical Examination

History

Identifying Data: Patient's name; age, race, sex. List the patient's significant medical problems. Name of informant (patient, relative).

Chief Compliant: Reason given by patient for seeking medical care and the duration of the symptom.

History of Present Illness (HPI): Describe the course of the patient's illness, including when it began, character of the symptoms, location where the symptoms began; aggravating or alleviating factors; pertinent positives and negatives. Describe past illnesses or surgeries, and past diagnostic testing.

Past Medical History (PMH): Past diseases, surgeries, hospitalizations; medical problems; history of diabetes, hypertension, peptic ulcer disease, asthma, myocardial infarction, cancer. In children include birth history, prenatal history, immunizations, and type of feedings.

Developmental history (in pediatrics)

Medications:

Allergies: Penicillin, codeine?

Family History: Medical problems in family, including problems similar to patient's disorder. Asthma, coronary artery disease, heart failure, cancer, tuberculosis.

Social History: Alcohol, smoking, drug usage. Marital status, employment situation. Level of education.

Review of Systems (ROS):

    General: Weight gain or loss, loss of appetite, fever, chills, fatigue, night sweats.

    Skin: Rashes, skin discolorations.

    Head: Headaches, dizziness, masses, seizures.

    Eyes: Visual changes, visual field deficits.

    Ears: Tinnitus, vertigo, hearing loss.

    Nose: Nose bleeds, discharge, sinus diseases.

    Mouth and Throat: Dental disease, hoarseness, throat pain.

    Respiratory: Cough, shortness of breath, sputum (color).

    Cardiovascular: Chest pain, orthopnea, paroxysmal nocturnal dyspnea; dyspnea on exertion, claudication, edema, valvular disease.

    Gastrointestinal: Dysphagia, abdominal pain, nausea, vomiting, hematemesis, diarrhea, constipation, melena (black tarry stools), hematochezia (bright red blood per rectum).

    Genitourinary: Dysuria, frequency, hesitancy, hematuria, discharge.

Gynecological: Gravida/para, abortions, last menstrual period (frequency, duration), age of menarche, menopause; dysmenorrhea, contraception, vaginal bleeding, breast masses.

Endocrine: Polyuria, polydipsia, skin or hair changes, heat intolerance.

Musculoskeletal: Joint pain or swelling, arthritis, myalgias.

Skin and Lymphatics: Easy bruising, lymphadenopathy.

Neuropsychiatric: Weakness, seizures, memory changes, depression.

Physical Examination

General appearance: Note whether the patient looks "ill," well, or malnourished.

Vital Signs: Temperature, heart rate, respirations, blood pressure.

Skin: Rashes, scars, moles, capillary refill (in seconds).

Lymph Nodes: Cervical, supraclavicular, axillary, inguinal nodes; size, tenderness.

Head: Bruising, masses. Check fontanels in pediatric patients.

Eyes: Pupils equal round and react to light and accommodation (PERRLA); extra ocular movements intact (EOMI), and visual fields. Funduscopy (papilledema, arteriovenous nicking, hemorrhages, exudates); scleral icterus, ptosis.

Ears: Acuity, tympanic membranes (dull, shiny, intact, injected, bulging).

Mouth and Throat: Mucus membrane color and moisture; oral lesions, dentition, pharynx, tonsils.

Neck: Jugular venous distention (JVD) at a 45 degree incline, thyromegaly, lymphadenopathy, masses, bruits, abdominojugular reflux.

Chest: Equal expansion, tactile fremitus, percussion, auscultation, rhonchi, crackles, rubs, breath sounds, egophony, whispered pectoriloquy.

Heart: Point of maximal impulse (PMI), thrills (palpable turbulence); regular rate and rhythm (RRR), first and second heart sounds (S1, S2); gallops (S3, S4), murmurs (grade 1-6), pulses (graded 0-2+).

Breast: Dimpling, tenderness, lumps, nipple discharge; axillary masses.

Abdomen: Contour (flat, scaphoid, obese, distended); scars, bowel sounds, bruits, tenderness, masses, liver span by percussion; hepatomegaly, splenomegaly; guarding, rebound, percussion note (tympanic), costovertebral angle tenderness (CVAT), suprapubic tenderness.

Genitourinary: Inguinal masses, hernias, scrotum, testicles, varicoceles.

Pelvic Examination: Vaginal mucosa, cervical discharge, uterine size, masses, adnexal masses, ovaries.

Extremities: Joint swelling, range of motion, edema (grade 1-4+); cyanosis, clubbing, edema (CCE); pulses (radial, ulnar, femoral, popliteal, posterior tibial, dorsalis pedis; simultaneous palpation of radial and femoral pulses).

Rectal Examination: Sphincter tone, masses, fissures; test for occult blood, prostate (nodules, tenderness, size).

Neurological: Mental status and affect; gait, strength (graded 0-5); touch sensation, pressure, pain, position and vibration; deep tendon reflexes (biceps, triceps, patellar, ankle; graded 0-4+); Romberg test (ability to stand erect with arms outstretched and eyes closed).

Cranial Nerve Examination:

  I: Smell

  II: Vision and visual fields

  III, IV, VI: Pupil responses to light, extraocular eye movements, ptosis

  V: Facial sensation, ability to open jaw against resistance, corneal reflex.

  VII: Close eyes tightly, smile, show teeth

  VIII: Hears watch tic; Weber test (lateralization of sound when tuning fork is placed on top of head); Rinne test (air conduction last longer than bone conduction when tuning fork is placed on mastoid process)

  IX, X: Palette moves in midline when patient says "ah," speech

  XI: Shoulder shrug and turns head against resistance

  XII: Stick out tongue in midline

Labs: Electrolytes (sodium, potassium, bicarbonate, chloride, BUN, creatinine), CBC (hemoglobin, hematocrit, WBC count, platelets, differential); x-rays, ECG, urine analysis (UA), liver function tests (LFTs).

Assessment (Impression): Assign a number to each problem and discuss separately. Discuss differential diagnosis and give reasons that support the working diagnosis; give reasons for excluding other diagnoses.

Plan: Describe therapeutic plan for each numbered problem, including testing, laboratory studies, medications, and antibiotics.

Problem-Oriented Daily Progress Note

Problem List: List each problem separately (heart failure, pneumonia, hypokalemia). State hospital day number, post-operative day number, and antibiotic day number.

Subjective: Describe how the patient feels in the patient's own words; and give observations about the patient.

Objective: Vital signs, physical exam for each system, laboratory data.

Assessment: Evaluate each numbered problem, and discuss the progress of each problem.

Plan: For each problem, discuss any additional orders, changes in drug regimen or plans for discharge or transfer.

Procedure Note

A procedure note should be written in the chart when a procedure is performed. Procedure notes are brief operative notes.

Procedure Note

Date and time:
Procedure:
Indications:
Patient Consent: Document that the indications, risks and alternatives to the procedure were explained to the patient. Note that the patient was given the opportunity to ask questions and that the patient consented to the procedure in writing.
Lab tests: Relevant labs, such as the INR and CBC
Anesthesia: Local with 2% lidocaine
Description of Procedure: Briefly describe the procedure, including sterile prep, anesthesia method, patient position, devices used, anatomic location of procedure, and outcome.
Complications and Estimated Blood Loss (EBL):
Disposition: Describe how the patient tolerated the procedure.
Specimens: Describe any specimens obtained and labs tests which were ordered.

Discharge Note

The discharge note should be written in the patient's chart prior to discharge.

Discharge Note

Date/time:
Diagnoses:
Treatment: Briefly describe therapy provided during hospitalization, including antibiotic therapy, surgery, and cardiovascular drugs.
Studies Performed: Electrocardiograms, CT scan.
Discharge medications:
Follow-up Arrangements:

Prescription Writing

- Patient's name:
- Date:
- Drug name and preparation (eg, tablets size): Lasix 40 mg
- Quantity to dispense: #40
- Frequency of administration: Sig: 1 po qAM
- Refills: None
- Signature

Discharge Summary

Patient's Name and Medical Record Number:
Date of Admission:
Date of Discharge:
Admitting Diagnosis:
Discharge Diagnosis:
Attending or Ward Team Responsible for Patient:
Surgical Procedures, Diagnostic Tests, Invasive Procedures:
Brief History, Pertinent Physical Examination, and Laboratory Data:
   Describe the course of the patient's disease up until the time that the patient
   came to the hospital, including physical exam and laboratory data.
Hospital Course: Describe the course of the patient's illness while in the
   hospital, including evaluation, treatment, medications, and outcome of
   treatment.
Discharged Condition: Describe improvement or deterioration in the patient's
   condition, and describe present status of the patient.
Disposition: Describe the situation to which the patient will be discharged
   (home, nursing home), and indicate who will take care of patient.
Discharged Medications: List medications and instructions for patient on
   taking the medications.
Discharged Instructions and Follow-up Care: Date of return for follow-up
   care at clinic; diet, exercise.
Problem List: List all active and past problems.
Copies: Send copies to attending, clinic, consultants.

10 Discharge Summary

Cardiovascular Disorders

Chest Pain and Myocardial Infarction

History of the Present Illness: Duration of chest pain. Location, radiation (to arm, jaw, back), character (squeezing, sharp, dull), intensity, rate of onset (gradual or sudden); relationship of pain to activity (at rest, during sleep, during exercise); relief by nitroglycerine; increase in frequency or severity of baseline anginal pattern. Improvement or worsening of pain.

Associated Symptoms: Diaphoresis, nausea, vomiting, dyspnea, orthopnea, edema, palpitations, dysphagia, cough, sputum, paresthesias, syncope.

Aggravating and Relieving Factors: Effect of inspiration on pain; effect of eating, NSAIDS, alcohol, stress.

Cardiac Testing: Past stress testing, angiograms, nuclear scans, ECGs.

Risk Factors for Coronary Heart Disease: Family history of coronary artery disease before age 55, diabetes, hypertension, smoking, hypercholesterolemia.

PMH: History of diabetes, claudication, stroke. Exercise tolerance; history of peptic ulcer disease. Prior history of myocardial infarction, coronary bypass grafting or angioplasty.

Social History: Cocaine usage, elicit drugs, smoking, alcohol.

Medications: Aspirin, beta-blockers, estrogen replacement, nicotine replacement therapy.

Physical Examination

General: Visible pain, apprehension, distress, pallor. Note whether the patient looks "ill," well, or malnourished.

Vital Signs: Pulse (tachycardia), BP, respirations (tachypnea), temperature.

Skin: Cold extremities (peripheral vascular disease), xanthomas (hypercholesterolemia).

HEENT: Fundi, "silver wire" arteries, arteriolar narrowing, A-V nicking, hypertensive retinopathy; carotid bruits, jugular venous distention.

Chest: Crackles, percussion note.

Heart: Decreased intensity of first heart sound (S1) (LV dysfunction); third heart sound (S3) (heart failure, dilation), S4 gallop (more audible in the left lateral position; decreased LV compliance due to ischemia); mitral insufficiency murmur (papillary muscle dysfunction), cardiac rub (pericarditis).

Abdomen: Epigastric tenderness (peptic ulcer), hepatomegaly, ascites, pulsatile mass (aortic aneurysm).

Rectal: Occult blood.

Extremities: Edema, femoral bruits, unequal or diminished pulses (aortic dissection); calf pain, swelling (thrombosis).

Labs:

Electrocardiographic Findings in Acute Myocardial Infarction: ST segment elevations in two contiguous leads with ST depressions in reciprocal leads, hyperacute T waves.

Chest x-ray: Cardiomegaly, pulmonary edema (CHF).

LDH, magnesium, CBC, electrolytes. CPK with isoenzymes, troponin I or troponin T, myoglobin, and LDH. Echocardiography.

Differential Diagnosis of Chest Pain

    A. **Acute Pericarditis.** Characterized by pleuritic-type chest pain and diffuse ST segment elevation.

    B. **Aortic Dissection.** "Tearing" chest pain with uncontrolled hypertension, widened mediastinum and increased aortic prominence on chest x-ray.

    C. **Esophageal Rupture.** Occurs after vomiting; x-ray may reveal air in mediastinum or a left side hydrothorax.

    D. **Acute Cholecystitis.** Characterized by right subcostal abdominal pain with anorexia, nausea, vomiting, and fever.

    E. **Acute Peptic Ulcer Disease.** Epigastric pain with melena or hematemesis, and anemia.

Dyspnea

History of the Present Illness: Rate of onset of shortness of breath (gradual, sudden), orthopnea (dyspnea when supine), paroxysmal nocturnal dyspnea (PND), chest pain, palpitations. Affect of physical exertion; history of myocardial infarction, syncope. Past episodes; aggravating or relieving factors (noncompliance with medications, salt overindulgence). Edema, weight gain, lightheadedness, cough, sputum, fever, anxiety; leg pain (DVT).

Past Medical History: Emphysema, heart failure, hypertension, occupational exposures, coronary artery disease, HIV risk factors, asthma.

Medications: Bronchodilators, cardiac medications (noncompliance), drug allergies.

Past Treatment or Testing: Cardiac testing, x-rays, ECG's, spirometry.

Physical Examination

General Appearance: Respiratory distress, dyspnea, pallor, diaphoresis. Note whether the patient looks "ill," well, or malnourished. Fluid input and output balance.

Vital Signs: BP (supine and upright), pulse (tachycardia), temperature, respiratory rate (tachypnea).

HEENT: Jugular venous distention at 45 degrees, tracheal deviation (pneumothorax).

Chest: Stridor (foreign body), retractions, breath sounds, wheezing, crackles (rales), rhonchi; dullness to percussion (pleural effusion), barrel chest (COPD); unilateral hyperresonance (pneumothorax).

Heart: Lateral displacement of point of maximal impulse; irregular, irregular rhythm (atrial fibrillation); S3 gallop (LV dilation), S4 (myocardial infarction), holosystolic apex murmur (mitral regurgitation); faint heart sounds (pericardial effusion).

Abdomen: Abdominojugular reflux (pressing on abdomen increases jugular vein distention), hepatomegaly, liver tenderness.

Extremities: Edema, pulses, cyanosis, clubbing. Calf tenderness or swelling (DVT).

Labs: ABG, cardiac enzymes; chest x-ray (cardiomegaly, hyperinflation with flattened diaphragms, infiltrates, effusions, pulmonary edema), ventilation/perfusion scan.

Electrocardiogram
   A. ST segment depression or elevation, new left bundle-branch block.
   B. ST elevations in two contiguous leads, with ST depressions in reciprocal leads (MI).

Differential Diagnosis: Heart failure, myocardial infarction, upper airway obstruction, pneumonia, pulmonary embolism, chronic obstructive pulmonary disease, asthma, pneumothorax, foreign body aspiration, hyperventilation, malignancy, anemia.

Edema

History of the Present Illness: Duration of edema; localized or generalized; associated pain, redness. History of heart failure, liver, or renal disease; weight changes, shortness of breath, malnutrition, chronic diarrhea (protein losing enteropathy), thyroid disease, prolonged immobility, allergies, alcoholism. Exacerbation by upright position.

Past Treating and Testing: Cardiac testing, chest x-rays. History of deep vein thrombosis, venous insufficiency. Recent fluid input and output balance.

Medications: Cardiac drugs, diuretics, calcium channel blockers.

Physical Examination

General Appearance: Respiratory distress, dyspnea, pallor, diaphoresis. Note whether the patient looks "ill," well, or malnourished.

Vitals: BP (orthostatic), pulse, temperature, respiratory rate.

HEENT: Jugular venous distention at 45°; carotid pulse amplitude.

Chest: Breath sounds, crackles, wheeze, dullness to percussion.

Heart: Displacement of point of maximal impulse, atrial fibrillation (irregular, irregular); S3 gallop (LV dilation), friction rubs.

Abdomen: Abdominojugular reflux, ascites, hepatomegaly, splenomegaly, distention, fluid wave, shifting dullness.

Extremities: Pitting or non-pitting edema (graded 1 to 4+), redness, warmth; mottled brown discoloration of ankle skin (venous insufficiency); leg circumference, tenderness, Homan's sign (dorsiflexion elicits pain; thrombosis); pulses, cyanosis, clubbing.

Labs: Electrolytes, liver function tests, CBC, chest x-ray, ECG, cardiac enzymes, Doppler studies of lower extremities.

Differential Diagnosis of Edema

Unilateral Edema: Deep venous thrombosis; lymphatic obstruction (neoplasm - pelvic, lymphoma).

Generalized Edema: Renal disease (acute glomerulonephritis, nephrotic syndrome, renal failure), heart failure, cirrhosis, obstruction of hepatic venous outflow, obstruction of inferior or superior vena cava.

Endocrine: Mineralocorticoid excess, hypoalbuminemia (protein losing enteropathy, malnutrition).

Miscellaneous: Chronic anemia, angioedema, iatrogenic edema.

Congestive Heart Failure

History of the Present Illness: Duration of dyspnea; note of onset (gradual, sudden); paroxysmal nocturnal dyspnea (PND), orthopnea; number of pillows needed under back when supine to prevent dyspnea; dyspnea on exertion (DOE); edema of lower extremities. Exercise tolerance (past and present), weight gain. Severity of dyspnea compared with past episodes.

Associated Symptoms: Fatigue, chest pain, pleuritic pain, cough, fever, chills, sputum, nausea, diaphoresis, palpitations, nocturia, syncope, viral illness.

Past Medical History: Past episodes of heart failure; hypertension, excess salt or fluid intake; noncompliance with diuretics, digoxin, antihypertensives; alcoholism, drug use, diabetes, coronary artery disease, myocardial infarction, heart murmur, arrhythmias. Thyroid disease, anemia, pulmonary disease.

Past Testing: Echocardiograms for ejection fraction, cardiac testing, angiograms, ECGs.

Cardiac Risk Factors: Smoking, diabetes, family history of coronary artery disease or heart failure, hypercholesterolemia, hypertension.

Precipitating Factors: Infections, noncompliance with low salt diet; excessive fluid intake; anemia, hyperthyroidism, pulmonary embolism, nonsteroidal antiinflammatory drugs, renal insufficiency; adverse drug reactions (beta blockers, calcium blockers, antiarrhythmics).

Treatment in Emergency Room: IV Lasix given, volume diuresed. Recent fluid input and output balance.

Physical Examination

General Appearance: Respiratory distress, anxiety, diaphoresis. Dyspnea, pallor. Note whether the patient looks "ill," well, or malnourished.

Vital Signs: BP (hypotension or hypertension), pulse (tachycardia), temperature, respiratory rate (tachypnea).

HEENT: Jugular venous distention at 45 degree incline (measure vertical distance from the sternal angle to top of column of blood); hepatojugular reflux (pressing on abdomen causes jugular venous distention); carotid pulse, amplitude, duration, bruits.

Chest: Breath sounds, crackles, rhonchi; dullness to percussion (pleural effusion).

Heart: Lateral displacement of point of maximal impulse; irregular, irregular rhythm (atrial fibrillation); S3 gallop (LV dilation).

Abdomen: Ascites, hepatomegaly, liver tenderness.

Extremities: Edema (graded 1 to 4+), pulses, jaundice, muscle wasting.

Labs: Chest x-ray: Cardiomegaly, perihilar congestion; vascular cephalization (increased density of upper lobe vasculature); Kerley B lines (horizontal streaks in lower lobes), pleural effusions.

ECG: Left ventricular hypertrophy, ectopic beats, atrial fibrillation.

Electrolytes, BUN, creatinine, sodium; CBC; serial cardiac enzymes, CPK, MB, troponins, LDH. Echocardiogram.

Conditions That Mimic or Provoke Heart Failure:

    A. Coronary artery disease and myocardial infarction

    B. Hypertension

    C. Aortic or mitral valve disease

    D. Cardiomyopathies: Hypertrophic, idiopathic dilated, postpartum, genetic, toxic, nutritional, metabolic

    E. Myocarditis: Infectious, toxic, immune

    F. Pericardial constriction

    G. Tachyarrhythmias or bradyarrhythmias

    H. Pulmonary embolism

    I. Pulmonary disease

    J. High output states: Anemia, hyperthyroidism, A-V fistulas, Paget's disease, fibrous dysplasia, multiple myeloma

    K. Renal failure, nephrotic syndrome

Factors Associated with Heart Failure

    A. Increase Demand: Anemia, fever, infection, excess dietary salt, renal failure, liver failure, thyrotoxicosis, AV fistula. Arrhythmias, cardiac ischemia/infarction, pulmonary emboli, alcohol abuse, hypertension.

    B. Medications: Antiarrhythmics (disopyramide), beta-blockers, calcium blockers, NSAID's, noncompliance with diuretics, excessive intravenous fluids

New York Heart Association Classification of Heart Failure

    Class I: Symptomatic only with strenuous activity.

Class II: Symptomatic with usual level of activity.
Class III: Symptomatic with minimal activity, but asymptomatic at rest.
Class IV: Symptomatic at rest.

Palpitations and Atrial Fibrillation

History of the Present Illness: Palpitations (rapid or irregular heart beat), fatigue, dizziness, nausea, dyspnea, edema; duration. Results of previous ECGs.

Associated Symptoms: Chest pain, pleuritic pain, syncope, weakness, fatigue, exercise intolerance, diaphoresis, symptoms of hyperthyroidism (tremor, anxiety).

Cardiac History: Hypertension, coronary disease, rheumatic heart disease, arrhythmias.

Underlying Conditions: Pneumonia, diabetes, noncompliance with cardiac medications, pericarditis, hyperthyroidism, electrolyte abnormalities, COPD, mitral valve stenosis, hypokalemia; diet pills, decongestants, alcohol, caffeine, cocaine.

Physical Examination

General Appearance: Respiratory distress, anxiety, diaphoresis. Dyspnea, pallor. Note whether the patient looks "ill," well, or malnourished.

Vital Signs: BP (hypotension), pulse (irregular, irregular tachycardia).

HEENT: Retinal hemorrhages, (emboli) jugular venous distention, carotid bruits; thyromegaly (hyperthyroidism).

Chest: Crackles (rales).

Heart: Irregular, irregular rhythm (atrial fibrillation); dyskinetic apical pulse, displaced point of maximal impulse (cardiomegaly), S4, mitral regurgitation murmur (rheumatic fever); pericardial rub (pericarditis).

Rectal: Occult blood.

Extremities: Peripheral pulses with irregular timing and amplitude. Edema, cyanosis, petechia (emboli). Femoral artery bruits (atherosclerosis).

Neuro: Motor weakness (embolic stroke), CN 2-12, sensory; dysphasia, dysarthria (stroke); tremor (hyperthyroidism).

Labs: Sodium, potassium, BUN, creatinine; magnesium; drug levels; CBC; serial cardiac enzymes; CPK, LDH, TSH, free T4. Chest x-ray.

ECG: Irregular R-R intervals with no P waves. Irregular baseline with rapid fibrillary waves (320 per minute). The ventricular response rate is 130-180 per minute.

Echocardiogram for atrial chamber size.

Differential Diagnosis of Atrial Fibrillation

　　Lone Atrial Fibrillation: No underlying disease state.

Cardiac Causes: Hypertensive heart disease with left ventricular hypertrophy, heart failure, mitral valve stenosis or regurgitation, pericarditis, hypertrophic cardiomyopathy, coronary artery disease, myocardial infarction, aortic stenosis, amyloidosis.

Noncardiac Causes: Hypoglycemia, theophylline intoxication, pneumonia, asthma, chronic obstructive pulmonary disease, pulmonary embolus, heavy alcohol intake or alcohol withdrawal, hyperthyroidism, systemic illness, electrolyte abnormalities. Stimulant abuse, excessive caffeine, over-the-counter cold remedies, illicit drugs.

Hypertension

History of the Present Illness: Degree of blood pressure elevation; patient's baseline BP from records; baseline BUN and creatinine. Age of onset of hypertension.

Associated Symptoms: Chest or back pain (aortic dissection), dyspnea, orthopnea, dizziness, blurred vision (hypertensive retinopathy); nausea, vomiting, headache (pheochromocytoma); lethargy, confusion (encephalopathy).

Paroxysms of tremor, palpitations, diaphoresis; edema, thyroid disease, angina; flank pain, dysuria, pyelonephritis. Alcohol withdrawal, noncompliance with antihypertensives (clonidine or beta-blocker withdrawal), excessive salt, alcohol.

Medications: Over-the-counter cold remedies, beta agonists, diet pills, ocular medications (sympathomimetics), bronchodilators, cocaine, amphetamines, nonsteroidal anti-inflammatory agents, oral contraceptives, cortico steroids.

Risk Factors for Coronary Artery Disease: Family history of coronary artery disease before age 55, diabetes, hypertension, smoking, hypercholesterolemia.

Past Testing: Urinalysis, ECG, creatinine.

Physical Examination

General Appearance: Delirium, confusion, agitation (hypertensive encephalopathy).

Vital Signs: Supine and upright blood pressure; BP in all extremities; pulse, temperature, respirations.

HEENT: Hypertensive retinopathy, hemorrhages, exudates, "cotton wool" spots, A-V nicking; papilledema; thyromegaly (hyperthyroidism). Jugular venous distention, carotid bruits.

Chest: Crackles (rales, pulmonary edema), wheeze, intercostal bruits (aortic coarctation).

Heart: Rhythm; laterally displaced, sustained, forceful, apical impulse with patient in left lateral position (ventricular hypertrophy); narrowly split S2 with increased aortic component; systolic ejection murmurs.

Abdomen: Renal bruits (bruit just below costal margin, renal artery stenosis); abdominal aortic enlargement (aortic aneurysm), renal masses, enlarged kidney (polycystic kidney disease); costovertebral angle tenderness. Truncal obesity (Cushing's syndrome).

Skin: Striae (Cushing's syndrome), uremic frost (chronic renal failure); hirsutism (adrenal hyperplasia); plethora (pheochromocytoma).

Extremities: Asymmetric femoral to radial pulses (coarctation of aortic); femoral bruits, edema (peripheral vascular disease); tremor (pheochromocytoma, hyperthyroidism).

Neuro: Mental status, rapid return phase of deep tendon reflexes (hyperthyroidism), localized weakness (stroke), visual acuity.

Labs: Potassium, BUN, creatinine, glucose, uric acid, CBC. UA with microscopic analysis (RBC casts, hematuria, proteinuria). 24 hour urine for metanephrines, plasma catecholamines (pheochromocytoma), plasma renin activity.

12 lead electrocardiography: Evidence of ischemic heart disease, rhythm and conduction disturbances, or left ventricular hypertrophy.

Chest x-ray: Cardiomegaly, indentation of aorta (coarctation), rib notching.

Findings Suggesting Secondary Hypertension:

    A. Primary Aldosteronism. Initial serum potassium <3.5 mEq/L while not taking medication.

    B. Aortic Coarctation. Femoral pulse delayed later than radial pulse; posterior systolic bruits below ribs.

    C. Pheochromocytoma. Tachycardia, tremor, pallor.

    D. Renovascular Stenosis. Paraumbilical abdominal bruits.

    E. Polycystic Kidneys. Flank or abdominal mass.

    F. Pyelonephritis. Urinary tract infections, costovertebral angle tenderness.

    G. Renal Parenchymal Disease. Increased serum creatinine ≥ 1.5 mg/dL, proteinuria.

Screening Tests for Secondary Hypertension	
Renovascular Hypertension	Captopril Test: Plasma renin level before and 1 hr after captopril 25 mg PO. A greater than 150% increase in renin is positive
	Captopril Renography: Renal scan before and after captopril 25 mg PO
	Intravenous pyelography
	MRI angiography
	Arteriography (DSA)

Hyperaldosteronism	Serum Potassium 24 hr urine potassium Plasma renin activity CT scan of adrenals
Pheochromocytoma	24 hr urine metanephrine Plasma catecholamine level CT scan Nuclear MIBG scan
Cushing's Syndrome	Plasma ACTH Dexamethasone suppression test
Hyperparathyroidism	Serum calcium Serum parathyroid hormone

Differential Diagnosis of Hypertension
A. **Primary (essential) Hypertension (90%)**
B. **Secondary Hypertension:** Renovascular hypertension, pheochromocytoma, cocaine use; withdrawal from alpha2 stimulants, clonidine or beta blockers, or alcohol; noncompliance with antihypertensive medications.

Pericarditis

History of the Present Illness: Sharp pleuritic chest pain; onset, intensity, radiation, duration. Exacerbated by supine position, coughing or deep inspiration; relieved by leaning forward; referred to trapezius ridge; fever, chills, palpitations, dyspnea.

Associated Findings: History of recent upper respiratory infection, autoimmune disease; prior episodes of pain; tuberculosis exposure; myalgias, arthralgias, rashes, fatigue, anorexia, weight loss, kidney disease.

Medications: Hydralazine, procainamide, isoniazid, penicillin.

Physical Examination

General Appearance: Respiratory distress, anxiety, diaphoresis. Dyspnea, pallor. Note whether the patient looks "septic," well, or malnourished.

Vital Signs: BP, pulse (tachycardia); pulsus paradoxus (drop in systolic BP >10 mmHg with inspiration).

HEENT: Cornea, sclera, iris lesions, oral ulcers (lupus); jugular venous distention (cardiac tamponade).

Skin: Malar rash (butterfly rash), discoid rash (lupus).

Chest: Crackles (rales), rhonchi.

Heart: Rhythm; friction rub on end-expiration while sitting forward; cardiac rub with 1-3 components at lower left sternal border; distant heart sounds (pericardial effusion).

Rectal: Occult blood.

Extremities: Arthralgias, joint tenderness.

Labs: ECG: diffuse, downwardly, concave, ST segment elevation in all 3 standard limb leads and several precordial leads; upright T waves, PR segment depression, low QRS voltage.

Chest x-ray: large cardiac silhouette; "water bottle sign;" pericardial calcifications.

Echocardiogram.

Increased WBC; UA, urine protein, urine RBCs; CPK, MB, LDH, blood culture, increased ESR.

Differential Diagnosis: Idiopathic pericarditis, infectious pericarditis (viral, bacterial, mycoplasmal, mycobacterial), Lyme disease, uremia, neoplasm, connective tissue disease, lupus, rheumatic fever, polymyositis, myxedema, sarcoidosis, post myocardial infarction pericarditis (Dressler's syndrome), drugs (penicillin, isoniazid, procainamide, hydralazine).

Syncope

History of the Present Illness: Time of occurrence and description of the episode. Duration of unconsciousness, rate of onset; activity before and after event. Body position, arm position (reaching), neck position (turning to side); mental status before and after event. Precipitants (fear, tension, hunger, pain, cough, micturition, defecation, exertion, Valsalva, hyperventilation, tight shirt collar).

Seizure activity (tonic/clonic). Chest pain, palpitations, dyspnea, weakness.

Prodromal Symptoms: Nausea, diaphoresis, pallor, lightheadedness, dimming vision (vasovagal syncope).

Post-syncopal disorientation, confusion, vertigo, flushing; urinary of fecal incontinence, tongue biting. Rate of return to alertness (delayed or spontaneous).

Past Medical History: History of past episodes of syncope, stroke, transient ischemic attacks, seizures, cardiac disease, arrhythmias, diabetes, anxiety attacks.

Past Testing: 24 hour Holter, exercise testing, cardiac testing, ECG, EEG.

Medications Associated with Syncope	
Antihypertensives or anti-angina agents	Antiarrhythmics
Adrenergic antagonists	Digoxin
Calcium channel blockers	Quinidine
Diuretics	Insulin
Nitrates	Drugs of abuse
Vasodilators	Alcohol
Antidepressants	Cocaine
Tricyclic antidepressants	Marijuana
Phenothiazines	

Physical Examination

General Appearance: Level of alertness, respiratory distress, anxiety, diaphoresis. Dyspnea, pallor. Note whether the patient looks "ill," well, or malnourished.

Vital Signs: Temperature, respiratory rate, postural vitals (supine and after standing 2-5 minutes), pulse. Blood pressure in all extremities; asymmetric radial to femoral artery pulsations (aortic dissection).

HEENT: Cranial bruising (trauma). Pupil size and reactivity, extraocular movements; tongue or buccal lacerations (seizure); flat jugular veins (volume depletion); carotid or vertebral bruits.

Skin: Turgor, capillary refill, pallor.

Chest: Crackles, rhonchi (aspiration).

Heart: Irregular rhythm (atrial fibrillation); systolic murmurs (aortic stenosis), cardiac friction rub.

Abdomen: Bruits, tenderness pulsatile mass.

Genitourinary/Rectal: Occult blood, urinary or fecal incontinence (seizure).

Extremities: Extremity palpation for trauma.

Neuro: Cranial nerves 2-12, strength, gait, sensory, mental status; nystagmus. Turn patient's head side to side, up and down; have patient reach above head, bend down and pick up object.

Labs: ECG: Arrhythmias, blocks. Chest x-ray, electrolytes, glucose, Mg, BUN, creatinine, CBC; 24-hour Holter monitor.

Differential Diagnosis of Syncope

Non-cardiovascular	Cardiovascular

Metabolic
  Hyperventilation
  Hypoglycemia
  Hypoxia
Neurologic
  Cerebrovascular insufficiency
  Normal pressure hydrocephalus
  Seizure
  Subclavian steal syndrome
  Increased intracranial pressure
Psychiatric
  Hysteria
  Major depression
	Reflex (heart structurally normal)
	  Vasovagal
	  Situational
	  Cough
	  Defecation
	  Micturition
	  Postprandial
	  Sneeze
	  Swallow
	  Carotid sinus syncope
	Orthostatic hypotension
	Drug-induced
	Cardiac
	  Obstructive
	  Aortic dissection
	  Aortic stenosis
	  Cardiac tamponade
	  Hypertrophic cardiomyopathy
	  Left ventricular dysfunction
	  Myocardial infarction
	  Myxoma
	  Pulmonary embolism
	  Pulmonary hypertension
	  Pulmonary stenosis
	  Arrhythmias
	    Bradyarrhythmias
	      Sick sinus syndrome
	      Pacemaker failure
	    Supraventricular and ventricular
	      tachyarrhythmias

Pulmonary Disorders

Hemoptysis

History of the Present Illness: Quantify the amount of blood, acuteness of onset, color (bright red, dark), character (coffee grounds, clots); dyspnea, chest pain (left or right), fever, chills; past bronchoscopies, exposure to tuberculosis; hematuria, weight loss, anorexia, malaise, hoarseness.

Farm exposure, homelessness, residence in a nursing home, immigration from a foreign country. Smoking, leg pain or swelling (pulmonary embolism), bronchitis, COPD, heart failure, anticoagulants, aspirin, NSAIDs, HIV risk factors (pulmonary Kaposi's sarcoma), aspiration of food or foreign body.

Family history of bleeding disorders.

Prior chest X-rays, CT scans, tuberculin testing (PPD).

Physical Examination

General Appearance: Dyspnea, respiratory distress. Anxiety, diaphoresis, pallor. Note whether the patient looks "ill," well, or malnourished.

Vital Signs: Temperature, respiratory rate (tachypnea), pulse (tachycardia), BP (hypotension); assess hemodynamic status.

HEENT: Nasal or oropharyngeal lesions, tongue lacerations; telangiectasias on buccal mucosa (Rendu-Osler-Weber disease); ulcerations of nasal septum (Wegener's granulomatosis), jugular venous distention, gingival disease (aspiration).

Lymph Nodes: Cervical, scalene or supraclavicular adenopathy (Virchow's nodes, intrathoracic malignancy).

Chest: Stridor, tenderness of chest wall; rhonchi, apical crackles (tuberculosis); localized wheezing (foreign body, malignancy), basilar crackles (pulmonary edema), pleural friction rub, breast masses (metastasis).

Heart: Mitral stenosis murmur (diastolic rumble), right ventricular gallop; accentuated, second heart sound (pulmonary embolism).

Abdomen: Masses, liver nodules (metastases), tenderness.

Extremities: Petechiae, ecchymoses (coagulopathy); cyanosis, tenderness, calf swelling (pulmonary embolism); clubbing (pulmonary disease), edema, bone pain (metastasis).

Rectal: Occult blood.

Skin: Purple plaques (Kaposi's sarcoma); rashes (paraneoplastic syndromes).

Labs: Sputum Gram stain, cytology, acid fast bacteria stain; CBC, platelets, ABG; pH of expectorated blood (alkaline=pulmonary; acidic=GI); UA (hematuria); INR/PTT, bleeding time; creatinine, sputum fungal culture; anti-glomerular basement membrane antibody, antinuclear antibody; PPD, cryptococcus antigen.

EKG, chest x-ray, CT scan, bronchoscopy, ventilation/perfusion scan.

Differential Diagnosis

    Infection: Bronchitis, pneumonia, lung abscess, tuberculosis, fungal infection, bronchiectasis, broncholithiasis.

    Neoplasms: Bronchogenic carcinoma, metastatic cancer, Kaposi's sarcoma.

    Vascular: Pulmonary embolism, mitral stenosis, pulmonary edema.

    Miscellaneous: Trauma, foreign body, aspiration, coagulopathy, epistaxis, oropharyngeal bleeding, vasculitis, Goodpasture's syndrome, lupus, hemosiderosis, Wegener's granulomatosis, pulmonary aneurysm rupture.

Wheezing and Asthma

History of the Present Illness: Onset, duration, and progression of wheezing; severity of attack compared to previous episodes; dyspnea, cough, fever, chills, purulent sputum; frequency of exacerbations and hospitalizations; history of steroid dependency, intubation, home oxygen or nebulizer use; baseline peak flow rate.

Exposure to allergens (foods, pollen, animals, drugs); seasons that provoke symptoms; exacerbation by exercise, aspirin, beta- blockers, new medications, recent upper respiratory infection; chest pain, foreign body aspiration.

Treatment given in emergency room and response.

Past Pulmonary History: Previous episodes of asthma, COPD, pneumonia, smoking. Baseline arterial blood gas results; past pulmonary function testing.

Family History: Family history of asthma, allergies, hay-fever, atopic dermatitis.

Physical Examination

General Appearance: Dyspnea, respiratory distress, diaphoresis, somnolence. Anxiety, diaphoresis, pallor. Note whether the patient looks cachectic, well, or malnourished.

Vital Signs: Temperature, respiratory rate (tachypnea >28/min), pulse (tachycardia), BP (widened pulse pressure, hypotension), pulsus paradoxus (inspiratory drop in systolic blood pressure >10 mmHg = severe attack).

HEENT: Nasal flaring, pharyngeal erythema, cyanosis, jugular venous distention, grunting.

Chest: Prolonged expiratory wheeze, rhonchi, decreased intensity of breath sounds (emphysema); sternocleidomastoid muscle contractions, barrel chest, increased anteroposterior diameter (hyperinflation); intracostal and supraclavicular retractions.

Heart: Decreased cardiac dullness to percussion (hyperinflation); distant heart sounds, third heart sound gallop (S3, cor pulmonale); increased intensity of pulmonic component of second heart sound (pulmonary hypertension).

Abdomen: Retractions, tenderness.

Extremities: Cyanosis, clubbing, edema.

Skin: Rash, urticaria.

Neuro: Decreased mental status, confusion.

Labs: Chest x-ray: hyperinflation, bullae, flattening of diaphragms; small, elongated heart.

ABG: Respiratory alkalosis, hypoxia.

Sputum gram stain; CBC, electrolytes, theophylline level.

ECG: Sinus tachycardia, right axis deviation, right ventricular hypertrophy. Pulmonary function tests, peak flow rate.

Differential Diagnosis: Asthma, bronchitis, COPD, pneumonia, congestive heart failure, anaphylaxis, upper airway obstruction, endobronchial tumors, carcinoid.

Chronic Obstructive Pulmonary Disease

History of the Present Illness: Duration of wheezing, dyspnea, cough, fever, chills; increased sputum production; sputum quantity, consistency, color; smoking (pack-years); chest trauma, noncompliance with medications. Severity of attack compared to prior episodes. Baseline blood gases.

Associated Symptoms: Chest pain, pleurisy. Adverse drug reactions (beta blockers, sedatives), allergic reaction.

Past History: Frequency of exacerbations, home oxygen use, steroid dependency, history of intubations, nebulizer use; pneumonia, past pulmonary function tests. Diabetes, heart failure, family history of emphysema, alcohol abuse.

Treatment given in emergency room.

Physical Examination

General Appearance: Diaphoresis, respiratory distress; speech interrupted by breaths. Anxiety, dyspnea, pallor. Note whether the patient looks "cachectic," well, or malnourished.

Vital Signs: Temperature, respiratory rate (tachypnea), pulse (tachycardia), BP.

HEENT: Pursed-lip breathing, jugular venous distention. Mucous membrane cyanosis, perioral cyanosis.

Chest: Barrel chest, retractions, sternocleidomastoid muscle contractions, supraclavicular retractions, intercostal retractions, prolonged expiratory wheezing, rhonchi. Decreased air movement, hyperinflation.

Heart: Right ventricular heave, distant heart sounds, S3 gallop (cor pulmonale).

Extremities: Cyanosis, clubbing, edema.

Neuro: Decreased mental status, somnolence, confusion.

Labs: Chest x-ray: Diaphragmatic flattening, bullae, hyperaeration.
ABG: Respiratory alkalosis (early), acidosis (late), hypoxia. Sputum gram stain, culture, CBC, electrolytes.
ECG: Sinus tachycardia, right axis deviation, right ventricular hypertrophy, PVCs.
Differential Diagnosis: COPD, chronic bronchitis, asthma, pneumonia, heart failure, alpha-1-antitrypsin deficiency, cystic fibrosis.

Pulmonary Embolism

History of the Present Illness: Sudden onset of pleuritic chest pain and dyspnea. Unilateral leg pain, swelling; fever, cough, hemoptysis, diaphoresis, syncope. History of deep vein thrombosis.
Virchow's Triad: Immobility, trauma, hypercoagulability; malignancy (pancreas, lung, genitourinary, stomach, breast, pelvic, bone); estrogens (oral contraceptives), history of heart failure, surgery, pregnancy.

Physical Examination

General Appearance: Dyspnea, apprehension, diaphoresis. Note whether the patient looks "cachectic," well, or malnourished.

Vitals: Temperature (fever), respiratory rate (tachypnea, >16/min), pulse (tachycardia >100/min), BP (hypotension).

HEENT: Jugular venous distention, prominent jugular A-waves.

Chest: Crackles; tenderness or splinting of chest wall, pleural friction rub; breast mass (malignancy).

Heart: Right ventricular gallop; accentuated, loud, pulmonic component of second heart sound (S2); S3 or S4 gallop; murmur.

Extremities: Cyanosis, edema, calf redness or tenderness; Homan's Sign (pain with dorsiflexion of foot); calf swelling, increased calf circumference (>2 cm difference), dilated superficial veins.

Rectal: Occult blood.

Genitourinary: Testicular or pelvic masses.

Neuro: Altered mental status.

Frequency of Symptoms and Signs in Pulmonary Embolism			
Symptoms	**%**	**Signs**	**%**
Dyspnea	84	Tachypnea (>16/min)	92
Pleuritic chest pain	74	Rales	58
Apprehension	59	Accentuated S2	53
Cough	53	Tachycardia	44
Hemoptysis	30	Fever (>37.8°C)	43
Sweating	27	Diaphoresis	36
Non-pleuritic chest pain	14	S3 or S4 gallop	34
Syncope	13	Thrombophlebitis	32

Labs: ABG: Hypoxemia, hypocapnia, respiratory alkalosis.

Lung Scan: Ventilation/perfusion mismatch. Duplex imaging and impedance plethysmography of lower extremities.

Pulmonary angiogram: Arterial filling defects.

Chest x-ray: Elevated hemidiaphragm, wedge shaped infiltrate; localized oligemia; effusion, segmental atelectasis.

ECG: Sinus tachycardia, nonspecific ST-T wave changes, QRS changes (acute right shift, S_1Q_3 pattern); right heart strain pattern (P-pulmonale, right bundle branch block, right axis deviation).

Differential Diagnosis: Heart failure, myocardial infarction, pneumonia, pulmonary edema, chronic obstructive pulmonary disease, asthma, aspiration of foreign body or gastric contents, hyperventilation.

Infectious Diseases

Fever and Sepsis

History of the Present Illness: Degree of fever; time of onset, pattern of fever; shaking chills (rigors), cough, sputum, sore throat, headache, neck stiffness, dysuria, frequency, back pain; night sweats; vaginal discharge, myalgias, nausea, vomiting, diarrhea, malaise, anorexia.

Chest or abdominal pain; ear, bone or joint pain; recent antipyretic use. Cirrhosis, diabetes, heart murmur, recent surgery; AIDS risk factors.

Exposure to tuberculosis or hepatitis; travel history, animal exposure; recent dental GI procedures. Ill contacts; IV or Foley catheter; antibiotic use, alcohol use, allergies.

Physical Examination

General Appearance: Lethargy, toxic appearance, altered level of consciousness. Dyspnea, apprehension, diaphoresis. Note whether the patient looks "ill," well, or malnourished.

Vital Signs: Temperature (fever curve), respiratory rate (tachypnea or hypoventilation), pulse (tachycardia), BP (hypotension).

HEENT: Papilledema; periodontitis, tympanic membrane inflammation, sinus tenderness; pharyngeal erythema, lymphadenopathy, neck rigidity.

Breast: Tenderness, masses.

Chest: Rhonchi, crackles, dullness to percussion (pneumonia).

Heart: Murmurs (endocarditis).

Abdomen: Masses, liver tenderness, hepatomegaly, splenomegaly; Murphy's sign (right upper quadrant tenderness and arrest of respiration secondary to pain, cholecystitis); shifting dullness, ascites. Costovertebral angle or suprapubic tenderness.

Extremities: Cellulitis, infected decubitus ulcers or wounds; IV catheter tenderness (phlebitis), calf tenderness, Homan's sign; joint or bone tenderness (septic arthritis). Osler's nodes, Janeway's lesions (peripheral lesions of endocarditis).

Rectal: Prostate tenderness; rectal flocculence, fissures, and anal ulcers.

Pelvic/Genitourinary: Cervical discharge, cervical motion tenderness; adnexal or uterine tenderness, adnexal masses; genital herpes lesions.

Skin: Pallor, cool extremities, delayed capillary refill; rash, purpura, petechia (septic emboli, meningococcemia), ecthyma gangrenosum (purpuric necrotic plaque of Pseudomonas infection). Pustules, cellulitis, furuncles, abscesses, cysts.

Labs: CBC, blood C&S x 2, glucose, BUN, creatinine, UA, urine Gram stain, C&S; lumbar puncture; urine, skin lesion cultures, bilirubin, transaminases;

tuberculin skin test, Gram Strain of buffy coat
Chest x-ray; abdomen X-ray; gallium, indium scans.

Laboratory Tests for Serious Infections	

Complete blood count, including leukocyte differential and platelet count
Electrolytes
Arterial blood gases
Blood urea nitrogen and creatinine
Urinalysis
INR, partial thromboplastin time, fibrinogen
Serum lactate
	Cultures with antibiotic sensitivities
	    Blood
	    Urine
	    Wound
	    Sputum, drains
	Chest X-ray
	Adjunctive imaging studies (eg, computed tomography, magnetic resonance imaging, abdominal X-ray)

Differential Diagnosis

Infectious Causes: Abscesses, mycobacterial infections (tuberculosis), cystitis, pyelonephritis, endocarditis, wound infection, diverticulitis, cholangitis, osteomyelitis, IV catheter phlebitis, sinusitis, otitis media, upper respiratory infection, pharyngitis, pelvic infection, cellulitis, hepatitis, infected decubitus ulcer, furuncle, peritonitis, abdominal abscess, perirectal abscess, mastitis; viral, parasite infections.

Malignancies: Lymphomas, leukemia, solid tumors, carcinomas.

Connective Tissue Diseases: Lupus, rheumatic fever, rheumatoid arthritis, temporal arteritis, sarcoidosis, polymyalgia rheumatica.

Other Causes of Fever: Atelectasis, drug fever, pulmonary emboli, pericarditis, pancreatitis, factitious fever, alcohol withdrawal. Deep vein thrombosis, myocardial infarction, gout, porphyria, thyroid storm.

Medications Associated with Fever: Barbiturates, isoniazid, nitrofurantoin, penicillins, phenytoin, procainamide, sulfonamides.

Cough and Pneumonia

History of the Present Illness: Duration of cough, chills, rigors, fever; rate of onset of symptoms. Sputum color, quantity, consistency, blood; living situation (nursing home, homelessness). Recent antibiotic use.

Associated Symptoms: Pleuritic chest pain, dyspnea, sore throat, rhinorrhea, headache, stiff neck, ear pain; nausea, vomiting, diarrhea, myalgias, arthralgias.

Past Medical History: Previous pneumonia, intravenous drug abuse, AIDS risk factors. Diabetes, heart failure, COPD, asthma, immunosuppression, alcoholism, steroids; ill contacts, aspiration, smoking, travel history, exposure to tuberculosis, tuberculin testing. Pneumococcal vaccination.

Physical Examination

General Appearance: Respiratory distress, dehydration. Note whether the patient looks "ill," well, or malnourished.

Vital Signs: Temperature (fever), respiratory rate (tachypnea), pulse (tachycardia), BP.

HEENT: Tympanic membranes, pharyngeal erythema, lymphadenopathy, neck rigidity.

Chest: Dullness to percussion, tactile fremitus (increased sound conduction); rhonchi; end-inspiratory crackles; bronchial breath sounds with decreased intensity; whispered pectoriloquy (increased transmission of sound), egophony (E to A changes).

Extremities: Cyanosis, clubbing.

Neuro: Gag reflex, mental status.

Labs: CBC, electrolytes, BUN, creatinine, glucose; UA, ECG, ABG.

Chest x-ray: segmental consolidation, air bronchograms, atelectasis, effusion.

Sputum Gram stain: >25 WBC per low-power field, bacteria.

Differential Diagnosis: Pneumonia, heart failure, asthma, bronchitis, viral infection, pulmonary embolism, malignancy.

Etiologic Agents of Community Acquired Pneumonia

Age 5-40 (without underlying lung disease): Viral, mycoplasma pneumoniae, Chlamydia pneumoniae, Streptococcus pneumoniae, legionella.

>40 (no underlying lung disease): Streptococcus pneumonia, group A streptococcus, H. influenza.

>40 (with underlying disease): Klebsiella pneumonia, Enterobacteriaceae, Legionella, Staphylococcus aureus, Chlamydia pneumoniae.

Aspiration Pneumonia: Streptococcus pneumoniae, Bacteroides sp., anaerobes, Klebsiella, Enterobacter.

Pneumocystis Carinii Pneumonia and AIDS

History of the Present Illness: Progressive exertional dyspnea and inability to perform usual activities (climbing stairs). Fever, chills, insidious onset; CD4 lymphocyte count and HIV-RNA titer (viral load); duration of HIV positivity; prior episodes of PCP or opportunistic infection.

Dry nonproductive cough (or productive of white, frothy sputum), night sweats. Prophylactic trimethoprim/sulfamethoxazole treatment; antiviral therapy. Baseline and admission arterial blood gas.

Associated Symptoms: Headache, stiff neck, lethargy, fatigue, weakness, malaise, weight loss, diarrhea, visual changes. Oral lesions, odynophagia (painful swallowing), skin lesions.

Past Infectious Disease History: History of herpes simplex, toxoplasmosis, tuberculosis, hepatitis, mycobacterium avium complex, syphilis. Prior pneumococcal immunization. Mode of acquisition of HIV infection; sexual, substance use history (intravenous drugs), blood transfusion.

Medications: Antivirals, prescribed and alternative medications.

Physical Examination

General Appearance: Cachexia, respiratory distress, cyanosis. Note whether the patient looks "ill," well, or malnourished.

Vital Signs: Temperature (fever), respiratory rate (tachypnea), pulse (tachycardia), BP (hypotension).

HEENT: Herpetic lesions; oropharyngeal thrush, hairy leukoplakia; oral Kaposi's sarcoma (purple-brown macules); retinitis, hemorrhages, perivascular white spots, cotton wool spots (CMV retinitis); visual field deficits (toxoplasmosis.) Neck rigidity, lymphadenopathy.

Chest: Dullness, decreased breath sounds at bases; crackles.

Heart: Murmurs (IV drug users).

Abdomen: Right upper quadrant tenderness, hepatosplenomegaly.

Pelvic/Rectal: Candidiasis, anal herpetic lesions, ulcers, condyloma.

Dermatologic Stigmata of AIDS: Rashes, Kaposi's sarcoma (multiple purple nodules or plaques), seborrheic dermatitis, zoster, herpes, molluscum contagiosum; oral thrush.

Lymph Node Examination: Enlarged nodes.

Neuro: Confusion, disorientation (AIDS dementia complex, meningitis), motor, sensory, cranial nerves.

Labs: Chest x-ray: Diffuse, interstitial infiltrates.

ABG: hypoxia, increased Aa gradient. CBC, sputum gram stain, Pneumocystis immunofluorescent stain; CD4 count, HIV RNA titer, hepatitis surface antigen and antibody, electrolytes. Bronchoalveolar lavage, high resolution CT scan.

Differential Diagnosis: Pneumocystis carinii pneumonia, bacterial pneumonia, tuberculosis, Kaposi's sarcoma.

Meningitis

History of the Present Illness: Duration and degree of fever, chills, rigors; headache, neck stiffness; cough, sputum; lethargy, irritability (high pitched cry in children), altered consciousness, nausea, vomiting. Skin rashes, dysuria, ill contacts, travel history.

History of pneumonia, bronchitis, otitis media, sinusitis, endocarditis. Diabetes, alcoholism, sickle cell disease, splenectomy malignancy, immunosuppression, AIDS, intravenous drug use, tuberculosis; recent upper respiratory infections, antibiotic use.

Physical Examination

General Appearance: Level of consciousness; obtundation, labored respirations. Note whether the patient looks "ill," well, or malnourished.

Vital Signs: Temperature (fever), pulse (tachycardia), respiratory rate (tachypnea), BP (hypotension).

HEENT: Pupil reactivity, extraocular movements, papilledema. Full fontanelle in infants. Brudzinski's sign (neck flexion causes hip flexion); Kernig's sign (flexing hip and extending knee elicits resistance).

Chest: Rhonchi, crackles.

Heart: Murmurs.

Skin: Capillary refill, rashes, nail bed splinter hemorrhages, Janeway's lesions (Endocarditis), petechia, purpura (meningococcemia).

Neuro: Altered mental status, cranial nerve palsies, weakness, sensory deficits, Babinski's sign.

CT Scan: Increased intracranial pressure should be excluded.

Labs

CSF Tube 1 - Gram stain, culture and sensitivity, bacterial antigen screen (1-2 mL).

CSF Tube 2 - Glucose, protein (1-2 mL).

CSF Tube 3 - Cell count and differential (1-2 mL).

CBC, electrolytes, BUN, creatinine.

Differential Diagnosis: Meningitis, encephalitis, brain abscess, viral infection, tuberculosis, osteomyelitis, subarachnoid hemorrhage.

Etiology of Bacterial Meningitis

15-50 years: Streptococcus pneumoniae, Neisseria meningitis, Listeria.

>50 years or debilitated: Same as above plus - Hemophilus influenza, Pseudomonas, streptococci.

AIDS: Cryptococcus neoformans, Toxoplasma gondii, herpes encephalitis, coccidioides.

Cerebral Spinal Fluid Analysis

Disease	Color	Protein	Cells	Glucose
Normal CSF Fluid	Clear	<50 mg/100 mL	<5 lymphs/mm^3	>40 mg/100 mL, ½-2/3 of blood glucose level drawn at same time
Bacterial meningitis or tuberculous meningitis	Yellow opalescent	Elevated 50-1500	25-10000 WBC with predominate polys	low
Tuberculous, fungal, partially treated bacterial, syphilitic meningitis, meningeal metastases	Clear opalescent	Elevated usually <500	10-500 WBC with predominant lymphs	20-40, low
Viral meningitis, partially treated bacterial meningitis, encephalitis, toxoplasmosis	Clear opalescent	Slightly elevated or normal	10-500 WBC with predominant lymphs	Normal to low

Pyelonephritis and Urinary Tract Infection

History of the Present Illness: Dysuria, frequency (voiding repeatedly of small amounts), urgency; suprapubic discomfort or pain, hematuria, fever, chills, malaise (pyelonephritis); back pain, nausea, vomiting.

History of urinary infections, renal stones or colicky pain. Recent antibiotic use, prostate enlargement. Diaphragm use.

Risk factors: Diaphragm or spermicide use, sexual intercourse, elderly, anatomic abnormality, calculi, prostatic obstruction, urinary tract instrumentation. Urinary tract obstruction, catheterization.

Physical Examination

General Appearance: Signs of dehydration, septic appearance. Note whether the patient looks "ill," well, or malnourished.

Vital Signs: Temperature (fever), respiratory rate, pulse, BP.

Abdomen: Suprapubic tenderness, costovertebral angle tenderness, masses.

Pelvic/Genitourinary: Urethral or vaginal discharge, cystocele.

Rectal: Prostatic hypertrophy or tenderness (prostatitis).

Labs: UA with micro. Urine Gram stain, urine C&S. CBC with differential, SMA7.

Pathogens: E coli, Klebsiella, Proteus, Pseudomonas, Enterobacter, Staphylococcus saprophyticus, enterococcus, group B streptococcus, Chlamydia trachomatis.

Differential Diagnosis: Acute cystitis, pyelonephritis, vulvovaginitis, gonococcal or chlamydia urethritis, herpes, cervicitis, papillary necrosis, renal calculus, appendicitis, cholecystitis, pelvic inflammatory disease.

Endocarditis

History of the Present Illness: Fever, chills, night sweats, fatigue, malaise, weight loss; pain in fingers or toes (emboli); pleuritic chest pain; skin lesions; history of heart murmur, rheumatic heart disease, heart failure, prosthetic valve.

Recent dental or gastrointestinal procedure; intravenous drug use, recent intravenous catheterization; urinary tract infection; colonic disease, decubitus ulcers, wound infection. History of stroke.

Physical Examination

General Appearance: Septic appearance. Note whether the patient looks "ill," well, or malnourished.

Vitals: Temperature (fever), pulse (tachycardia), BP (hypotension).

HEENT: Oral mucosal and conjunctival petechiae; Roth's spots (retinal hemorrhages with pale center, emboli).

Heart: New or worsening cardiac murmur.

Abdomen: Liver tenderness (abscess); splenomegaly, spinal tenderness (vertebral abscess).

Neuro: Focal neurological deficits (septic emboli).

Extremities: Splinter hemorrhages under nails; Osler's nodes (erythematous or purple tender nodules on pads of toes or fingers); Janeway lesions (erythematous, nontender lesions on palms and soles, septic emboli), joint pain (septic arthritis).

Labs: WBC, UA (hematuria); blood cultures x 3, urine culture.

Echocardiogram: Vegetations, valvular insufficiency.

Chest x-ray: Cardiomegaly, valvular calcifications, multiple focal infiltrates.

Native Valve Pathogens: Streptococcus viridans, streptococcus bovis, enterococci, staphylococcus aureus, streptococcus pneumonia, pseudomonas, group D streptococcus.

Prosthetic Valve Pathogens: Staphylococcus aureus, Enterobacter sp., staphylococcus epidermidis.

Gastrointestinal Disorders

Abdominal Pain and the Acute Abdomen

History of the Present Illness: Duration of pain, pattern of progression; exact location at onset and at present; diffuse or localized; location and character at onset and at present (burning, crampy, sharp, dull); constant or intermittent ("colicky"); radiation (to shoulder, back, groin); sudden or gradual onset. Effect of eating, vomiting, defecation, flatus, urination, inspiration, movement, position. Timing and characteristics of last bowel movement. Similar episodes in past; relation to last menstrual period.

Associated Symptoms: Fever, chills, nausea, vomiting (bilious, feculent, undigested food, blood, coffee grounds); vomiting before or after onset of pain; jaundice, constipation, change in bowel habits or stool caliber, obstipation (inability to pass gas); chest pain, diarrhea, hematochezia (rectal bleeding), melena (black, tarry stools); dysuria, hematuria, anorexia, weight loss, dysphagia, odynophagia (painful swallowing); early satiety, trauma.

History of abdominal surgery (appendectomy, cholecystectomy, aortic graft), hernias, gallstones; coronary disease, kidney stones; alcoholism, cirrhosis, peptic ulcer, dyspepsia.

Past Treatment or Testing: Endoscopies, x-rays, upper GI series.

Aggravating or Relieving Factors: Fatty food intolerance, medications, aspirin, NSAID's, narcotics, anticholinergics, laxatives, antacids.

Physical Examination

General Appearance: Degree of distress, body positioning to relieve pain, nutritional status. Signs of dehydration, septic appearance. Note whether the patient looks "ill," well, or malnourished.

Vitals: Temperature (fever), pulse (tachycardia), BP (hypotension), respiratory rate (tachypnea).

HEENT: Pale conjunctiva, scleral icterus, atherosclerotic retinopathy, "silver wire" arteries (ischemic colitis); flat neck veins (hypovolemia). Lymphadenopathy, Virchow node (supraclavicular mass).

Abdomen

Inspection: Scars, ecchymosis, visible peristalsis (small bowel obstruction), distension. Scaphoid, flat.

Auscultation: Absent bowel sounds (paralytic ileus or late obstruction), high-pitched rushes (obstruction), bruits (ischemic colitis).

Palpation: Begin palpation in quadrant diagonally opposite to point of maximal pain with patient's legs flexed and relaxed. Bimanual palpation of flank (renal disease or retrocecal appendix). Rebound tenderness; hepatomegaly, splenomegaly, masses; hernias (incisional, inguinal, femoral). Pulsating masses; costovertebral angle tenderness. Bulging flanks, shifting dullness, fluid wave (ascites).

Specific Signs on Palpation

Murphy's sign: Inspiratory arrest with right upper quadrant palpation, cholecystitis.

Charcot's sign: Right upper quadrant pain, jaundice, fever; gallstones.

Courvoisier's sign: Palpable, nontender gallbladder with jaundice; pancreatic malignancy.

McBurney's point tenderness: Located two thirds of the way between umbilicus and anterior superior iliac spine; appendicitis.

Iliopsoas sign: Elevation of legs against examiner's hand causes pain, retrocecal appendicitis. Obturator sign: Flexion of right thigh and external rotation of thigh causes pain in pelvic appendicitis.

Rovsing's sign: Manual pressure and release at left lower quadrant colon causes referred pain at McBurney's point; appendicitis.

Cullen's sign: Bluish periumbilical discoloration; peritoneal hemorrhage.

Grey Turner's sign: Flank ecchymoses; retroperitoneal hemorrhage.

Percussion: Loss of liver dullness (perforated viscus, free air in peritoneum); liver and spleen span by percussion.

Rectal Examination: Masses, tenderness, impacted stool; gross or occult blood.

Genital/Pelvic Examination: Cervical discharge, adnexal tenderness, uterine size, masses, cervical motion tenderness.

Extremities: Femoral pulses, popliteal pulses (absent pulses indicate ischemic colitis), edema.

Skin: Jaundice, dependent purpura (mesenteric infarction), petechia (gonococcemia).

Stigmata of Liver Disease: Spider angiomata, periumbilical collateral veins (Caput medusae), gynecomastia, ascites, hepatosplenomegaly, testicular atrophy.

Labs: CBC, electrolytes, liver function tests, amylase, lipase, UA, pregnancy test. ECG.

Chest x-ray: Free air under diaphragm, infiltrates, effusion (pancreatitis).

X-rays of abdomen (acute abdomen series): Flank stripe, subdiaphragmatic free air, distended loops of bowel, sentinel loop, air fluid levels, thumb printing, mass effects, calcifications, fecaliths, portal vein gas, pneumatobilia.

Differential Diagnosis

Generalized Pain: Intestinal infarction, peritonitis, obstruction, diabetic ketoacidosis, sickle crisis, acute porphyria, penetrating posterior duodenal ulcer, psychogenic pain.

Right Upper Quadrant: Cholecystitis, cholangitis, hepatitis, gastritis, pancreatitis, hepatic metastases, gonococcal perihepatitis (Fitz-Hugh-Curtis syndrome), retrocecal appendicitis, pneumonia, peptic ulcer.

Epigastrium: Gastritis, peptic ulcer, gastroesophageal reflux disease, esophagitis, gastroenteritis, pancreatitis, perforated viscus, intestinal obstruction, ileus, myocardial infarction, aortic aneurysm.

Left Upper Quadrant: Peptic ulcer, gastritis, esophagitis, gastroesophageal reflux, pancreatitis, myocardial ischemia, pneumonia, splenic infarction, pulmonary embolus.

Left Lower Quadrant: Diverticulitis, intestinal obstruction, colitis, strangulated hernia, inflammatory bowel disease, gastroenteritis, pyelonephritis, nephrolithiasis, mesenteric lymphadenitis, mesenteric thrombosis, aortic aneurysm, volvulus, intussusception, sickle crisis, salpingitis, ovarian cyst, ectopic pregnancy, endometriosis, testicular torsion, psychogenic pain.

Right Lower Quadrant: Appendicitis, diverticulitis (redundant sigmoid) salpingitis, endometritis, endometriosis, intussusception, ectopic pregnancy, hemorrhage or rupture of ovarian cyst, renal calculus.

Hypogastric/Pelvic: Cystitis, salpingitis, ectopic pregnancy, diverticulitis, strangulated hernia, endometriosis, appendicitis, ovarian cyst torsion; bladder distension, nephrolithiasis, prostatitis, malignancy.

Nausea and Vomiting

History of the Present Illness: Character of emesis (color, food, bilious, feculent, hematemesis, coffee ground material, projectile); abdominal pain, effect of vomiting on pain; early satiety, fever, melena, vertigo, tinnitus (labyrinthitis).

Clay colored stools, dark urine, jaundice (biliary obstruction); recent change in medications. Ingestion of spoiled food ; exposure to Ill contacts; dysphagia, odynophagia.

Possibility of pregnancy (last menstrual period, contraception, sexual history). Diabetes, cardiac disease, peptic ulcer, liver disease, CNS disease, headache.

Drugs Associated with Nausea: Digoxin, colchicine, theophylline, chemotherapy, anticholinergics, morphine, meperidine (Demerol), ergotamines, oral contraceptives, progesterone, antiarrhythmics, erythromycin, antibiotics, antidepressants.

Past Testing: X-rays, upper GI series, endoscopy.

Physical Examination

General Appearance: Signs of dehydration, septic appearance. Note whether the patient looks "ill," well, or malnourished.

Vital Signs: BP (orthostatic hypotension), pulse (tachycardia), respiratory rate, temperature (fever).

Skin: Pallor, jaundice, spider angiomas.

HEENT: Nystagmus, papilledema; ketone odor on breath (apple odor, diabetic ketoacidosis); jugular venous distention or flat neck veins.

Abdomen: Scars, bowel sounds, bruits, tenderness, rebound, rigidity, distention, hepatomegaly, ascites.

Extremities: Edema.

Rectal: Masses, occult blood.

Labs: CBC, electrolytes, UA, amylase, lipase, LFTs, pregnancy test, four views of the abdomen series.

Differential Diagnosis: Gastroenteritis, systemic infections, medications (contraceptives, antiarrhythmics, chemotherapy, antibiotics), pregnancy, appendicitis, peptic ulcer, cholecystitis, hepatitis, intestinal obstruction, gastroesophageal reflux, gastroparesis, ileus, pancreatitis, myocardial ischemia, tumors (esophageal, gastric) increased intracranial pressure, labyrinthitis, diabetic ketoacidosis, renal failure, toxins, bulimia, psychogenic vomiting.

Anorexia and Weight Loss

History of the Present Illness: Time of onset, amount and rate of weight loss (sudden, gradual); change in appetite, nausea, vomiting, dysphagia, abdominal pain; exacerbation of pain with eating (intestinal angina); diarrhea, fever, chills, night sweats; dental problems; restricted access to food.

Polyuria, polydipsia; skin or hair changes; 24-hour diet recall; dyspepsia, jaundice, dysuria; cough, change in bowel habits; chronic medical illness.

Dietary restrictions (low salt, low fat); diminished taste, malignancy, AIDS risks factors; psychiatric disease, renal disease, alcoholism, drug abuse (cocaine, amphetamines).

Signs of depression: Weight change, change in appetite, loss of interest in usual activities, sleep abnormalities, decreased libido.

Physical Examination

General Appearance: Muscle wasting, cachexia. Signs of dehydration. Note whether the patient looks "ill," well, or malnourished.

Vital Signs: Pulse (bradycardia), BP, respiratory rate, temperature (hypothermia).

Skin: Pallor, jaundice, hair changes, skin laxity, cheilosis, dermatitis, glossitis (Pellagra).

HEENT: Dental erosions from vomiting, oropharyngeal lesions, thyromegaly, glossitis, temporal wasting, supraclavicular adenopathy (Virchow's node).

Chest: Rhonchi, barrel shaped chest.

Heart: Murmurs, displaced PMI.

Abdomen: Scars, decreased bowel sounds, tenderness, hepatomegaly splenomegaly. Periumbilical adenopathy, palpable masses.

Extremities: Edema, muscle wasting, lymphadenopathy, skin abrasions on fingers.

Neuropathy: Decreased sensation, poor proprioception.

Rectal: Occult blood, masses.

Labs: CBC, electrolytes, protein, albumin, pre-albumin, transferrin, thyroid studies, LFTs, toxicology screen.

Differential Diagnosis: Inadequate caloric intake, peptic ulcer, depression, anorexia nervosa, dementia, hyper/hypothyroidism, cardiopulmonary disease, narcotics, diminished taste, diminished olfaction, poor dental hygiene (loose dentures), cholelithiasis, malignancy (gastric carcinoma), gastritis, hepatic or renal failure, systemic infection, alcohol abuse, AIDS, mesenteric ischemia.

Diarrhea

History of the Present Illness: Rate of onset, duration, frequency, timing of the diarrheal episodes. Volume of stool output (number of stools per day), watery stools; fever. Cramping, abdominal cramps, bloating, flatulence, tenesmus (painful urge to defecate), anorexia, nausea, vomiting, bloating; lightheadedness, myalgias, arthralgias, weight loss.

Stool Appearance: Buoyancy, blood or mucus, oily, foul odor.

Recent ingestion of spoiled poultry (salmonella), milk, seafood (shrimp, shellfish; Vibrio parahaemolyticus); common sources (restaurant), travel history, laxative abuse.

Ill contacts with diarrhea; inflammatory bowel disease, hyperthyroidism; family history of coeliac disease.

Sexual exposures, immunosuppressive agents, AIDS risk factors, coronary artery disease, peripheral vascular disease (ischemic colitis). Exacerbation by stress.

Drugs and Substances Associated with Diarrhea: Laxatives, magnesium-containing antacids, sulfa drugs, antibiotics (erythromycin, clindamycin), cholinergic agents, colchicine, milk (lactase deficiency), gum (sorbitol).

Physical Examination

General Appearance: Signs of dehydration or malnutrition. Septic appearance. Note whether the patient looks "ill," well, or malnourished.

Vital Signs: BP (orthostatic hypotension), pulse (tachycardia), respiratory rate, temperature (fever).

Skin: Skin turgor, delayed capillary refill, jaundice.

HEENT: Oral ulcers (inflammatory bowel or coeliac disease), dry mucous membranes, cheilosis (cracked lips, riboflavin deficiency); glossitis (B12, folate deficiency). Oropharyngeal candidiasis (AIDS).

Abdomen: Hyperactive bowel sounds, tenderness, rebound, hepatomegaly guarding, rigidity (peritoneal signs), distention, bruits (ischemic colitis).

Extremities: Arthritis, joint swelling (ulcerative colitis). Absent peripheral pulses or bruits (ischemic colitis).

Rectal: Perianal or rectal ulcers, sphincter tone, tenderness, masses, occult blood. Sphincter reflex.

Neuro: Mental status changes. Peripheral neuropathy (B6, B12 deficiency), decreased perianal sensation.

Labs: Electrolytes, Wright's stain for fecal leucocytes; cultures for enteric pathogens, ova and parasites x 3; clostridium difficile toxin. CBC with differential, calcium, albumen, flexible sigmoidoscopy.

Abdominal X-ray: Air fluid levels, dilation, pancreatic calcifications.

Differential Diagnosis

Acute Infectious Diarrhea: Infectious diarrhea (salmonella, shigella, E coli, Campylobacter, Bacillus cereus), enteric viruses (rotavirus, Norwalk virus), traveler's diarrhea, antibiotic-related diarrhea

Chronic Diarrhea:

Osmotic Diarrhea: Laxatives, lactulose, lactase deficiency (gastroenteritis, sprue), other disaccharidase deficiencies, ingestion of mannitol, enteral feeding, sorbitol.

Secretory Diarrhea: Bacterial enterotoxins, viral infection; AIDS associated disorders (mycobacterial, HIV), Zollinger-Ellison syndrome, vasoactive intestinal peptide tumor, carcinoid tumors, medullary thyroid carcinoma, colonic villus adenoma.

Exudative Diarrhea: Bacterial infection, Clostridium difficile, parasites, Crohn's disease, ulcerative colitis, diverticulitis, intestinal ischemia, diverticulitis.

Diarrhea Secondary to Altered Intestinal Motility: Diabetic gastroparesis, hyperthyroidism, laxatives, cholinergics, irritable bowel syndrome, "dumping syndrome," bacterial overgrowth, constipation-related diarrhea.

Hematemesis and Upper Gastrointestinal Bleeding

History of the Present Illness: Duration and frequency of hematemesis (bright red blood, coffee ground material), volume of blood, hematocrit. Forceful retching prior to hematemesis (Mallory-Weiss tear).

Abdominal pain, melena, hematochezia (bright red blood per rectum); history of peptic ulcer, esophagitis, prior bleeding episodes.

Ingestion of alcohol, aspirin, nonsteroidal anti-inflammatory drugs, steroids, anticoagulants; nose bleeds, syncope, lightheadedness, nausea.

Weight loss, malaise, fatigue, anorexia, early satiety, jaundice. History of liver or renal disease, hepatic encephalopathy, esophageal varices, aortic surgery.

Nasogastric aspirate quantity and character; transfusions given previously. Family history of liver disease or bleeding disorders.

Past Testing: X-ray studies, endoscopy.

Past Treatment: Endoscopic sclerotherapy, shunt surgery.

Physical Examination

General Appearance: Pallor, diaphoresis, cold extremities, confusion. Signs of dehydration. Note whether the patient looks "ill," well, or malnourished.

Vital Signs: Supine and upright pulse and blood pressure (orthostatic hypotension); (resting tachycardia indicates a 10% blood volume loss; postural hypotension indicates a 20-30% blood loss); oliguria (<20 mL of urine per hour), temperature.

Skin: Delayed capillary refill, pallor, petechiae. Stigmata of liver disease [jaundice, umbilical venous collaterals (caput medusae), spider angiomas, parotid gland hypertrophy]. Hemorrhagic telangiectasia (Osler-Weber-Rendu syndrome), abnormal pigmentation (Peutz-Jeghers syndrome); purple brown nodules (Kaposi's sarcoma).

HEENT: Scleral pallor, oral telangiectasia, flat neck veins.

Chest: Gynecomastia (cirrhosis), breast masses (metastatic disease).

Heart: Systolic ejection murmur.

Abdomen: Scars, tenderness, rebound, masses, splenomegaly, hepatic atrophy (cirrhosis), liver nodules. Ascites, dilated abdominal veins.

Extremities: Dupuytren's contracture (palmar contractures, cirrhosis), edema.

Neuro: Decreased mental status, confusion, poor memory, asterixis (flapping with wrists when hyperextended, hepatic encephalopathy).

Genitourinary/Rectal: Gross or occult blood, masses, testicular atrophy.

Labs: CBC, platelets, electrolytes, BUN (elevation suggests upper GI bleed), glucose, INR/PTT, ECG. Endoscopy, nuclear scan, angiography.

Differential Diagnosis of Upper GI Bleeding: Gastric or duodenal ulcer, esophageal varices, Mallory Weiss tear (gastroesophageal junction tear due to vomiting or retching), gastritis, esophagitis, swallowed blood (nose bleed, oral lesion), duodenitis, gastric cancer, vascular ectasias, coagulopathy, hypertrophic gastropathy (Menetrier's disease), aorto-enteric fistula.

Melena and Lower Gastrointestinal Bleeding

History of the Present Illness: Duration, quantity, color of bleeding (gross blood, streaks on stool, melena), recent hematocrit. Change in bowel habits or stool caliber, abdominal pain, fever. Constipation, diarrhea, anorectal pain. Epistaxis, anorexia, weight loss, malaise, vomiting.

Fecal mucus, tenesmus (straining during defecation), lightheadedness; history of diverticulosis, hemorrhoids, colitis, peptic ulcer, hematemesis, bleeding disease, coronary or renal disease, cirrhosis, alcoholism, easy bruising.

Anticoagulants, aspirin, NSAIDS.

Color of nasogastric aspirate.

Past Testing: Barium enema, colonoscopy, sigmoidoscopy, upper GI series.

Physical Examination

General Appearance: Signs of dehydration, pallor. Note whether the patient looks ill, well, or malnourished.

Vital Signs: BP, pulse (orthostatic hypotension), respiratory rate, temperature (tachycardia), oliguria.

Skin: Cold, clammy skin; delayed capillary refill, pallor, jaundice. Stigmata of liver disease: Umbilical venous collaterals (Caput medusae), jaundice, spider angiomata, parotid gland hypertrophy, gynecomastia. Rashes, purpura; buccal mucosa discolorations or pigmentation (Henoch-Schönlein purpura or Peutz-Jeghers polyposis syndrome).

HEENT: Atherosclerotic retinal disease, "silver wire" arteries (ischemic colitis).

Heart: Systolic ejection murmurs; atrial fibrillation (mesenteric emboli).

Abdomen: Scars, bruits, masses, distention, rebound, tenderness, hernias, liver atrophy (cirrhosis), splenomegaly. Ascites, pulsatile masses (aortic aneurysm).

Genitourinary: Testicular atrophy.

Extremities: Cold, pale extremities.

Neuro: Decreased mental status, confusion, asterixis (flapping hand tremor; hepatic encephalopathy).

Rectal: Gross or occult blood, masses, hemorrhoids; fissures, polyps, ulcers.

Labs: CBC (anemia), liver function tests. Abdominal x-ray series (thumbprinting, air fluid levels).

Differential Diagnosis of Lower Gastrointestinal Bleeding: Hemorrhoids, fissures, diverticulosis, upper GI bleeding, rectal trauma, inflammatory bowel disease, infectious or ischemic colitis, bleeding polyps, carcinoma, angiodysplasias, intussusception, coagulopathies, Meckel's diverticulitis, epistaxis, endometriosis, aortoenteric fistula.

Cholecystitis

History of the Present Illness: Duration of biliary colic (constant right upper quadrant pain, 30-90 minutes after meals, lasting several hours). Radiation to epigastrium, scapula or back; nausea, vomiting, anorexia, low grade fever; fatty food intolerance, dark urine, clay colored stools; bloating, jaundice, early satiety, flatulence, obesity.

Previous epigastric pain, gallstones, alcohol. History of fasting, rapid weight loss, hyperalimentation, estrogen, pregnancy, diabetes, sickle cell anemia, hereditary spherocytosis.

Prior Testing: Ultrasounds, HIDA scans, endoscopies.

Causes of Cholesterol Stones: Hereditary, pregnancy, exogenous steroids, diabetes, Crohn's disease, terminal ileal resection; rapid weight loss, hyperalimentation.

Causes of Pigment Stones: Asians with biliary parasites, sickle cell anemia, hereditary spherocytosis, cirrhosis, biliary stasis.

Physical Examination

General Appearance: Obese, restless patient unable to find a comfortable position. Signs of dehydration, septic appearance. Note whether the patient looks "ill," well, or malnourished.

Vital Signs: Pulse (mild tachycardia), temperature (low-grade fever), respiratory rate (shallow respirations), BP.

Skin: Jaundice

HEENT: Scleral icterus, sublingual jaundice.

Abdomen: Epigastric or right upper quadrant tenderness, Murphy's sign (tenderness and inspiratory arrest during palpation of RUQ); firm tender, sausage-like mass in RUQ (enlarged gallbladder); guarding, rigidity, rebound (peritoneal signs); Charcot's sign (intermittent right upper quadrant abdominal pain, jaundice, fever).

Labs: Ultrasound, HIDA (radionuclide) scan, WBC, hyperbilirubinemia, alkaline phosphatase, AST, amylase.

Plain Abdominal X-ray: Increased gallbladder shadow, gallbladder calcifications; air in gallbladder wall (emphysematous cholecystitis), small bowel obstruction (gallstone ileus).

Differential Diagnosis: Calculus cholecystitis, cholangitis, peptic ulcer, pancreatitis, appendicitis, gastroesophageal reflux disease, hepatitis, nephrolithiasis, pyelonephritis, hepatic metastases, gonococcal perihepatitis (Fitz-Hugh-Curtis syndrome), pleurisy, pneumonia, angina, herpes zoster.

Jaundice and Hepatitis

History of the Present Illness: Dull right upper quadrant pain, anorexia, jaundice, nausea, vomiting, fever, dark urine, increased abdominal girth (ascites), pruritus, arthralgias, urticarial rash; somnolence (hepatic encephalopathy). Weight loss, melena, hematochezia, hematemesis.

IV drug abuse, alcoholism, exposure to hepatitis or jaundiced persons, blood transfusion, day care centers, residential institutions, foreign travel history; prior hepatitis immunization. Heart failure, sepsis.

Hepatotoxins: Acetaminophen, isoniazid, nitrofurantoin, methotrexate, sulfonamides, NSAIDS, phenytoin.

Family history of jaundice/liver disease.

Prior Testing: Hepatitis serologies, liver function tests, liver biopsy.

Physical Examination

General Appearance: Signs of dehydration, septic appearance. Note whether the patient looks "ill," well, or malnourished.

Vital Signs: Pulse, BP, respiratory rate, temperature (fever).

Skin: Jaundice, needle tracks, sclerotic veins (from intravenous injections), urticaria, spider angiomas, bronze discoloration (hemochromatosis).

HEENT: Scleral icterus, sublingual jaundice, lymphadenopathy, Kayser-Fleischer rings (bronze corneal pigmentation, Wilson's disease).

Chest: Gynecomastia, Murphy's sign (cessation of inspiration with palpation of the right upper quadrant).

Abdomen: Scars, bowel sounds, right upper quadrant tenderness; liver span, hepatomegaly; liver margin texture (blunt, irregular, firm), splenomegaly (hepatitis) or hepatic atrophy (cirrhosis), ascites. Umbilical venous collaterals (Caput medusae). Courvoisier's sign (palpable nontender gallbladder with jaundice; pancreatic or biliary malignancy).

Genitourinary: Testicular atrophy.

Extremities: Joint tenderness, palmar erythema, Dupuytren's contracture (fibrotic palmar ridge).

Neuro: Disorientation, confusion, asterixis (flapping tremor when wrists are hyperextended, encephalopathy).

Rectal: Occult blood; hemorrhoids.

Labs: CBC with differential, LFTs, amylase, lipase, hepatitis serologies (hepatitis B surface antibody, hepatitis B surface antigen, hepatitis A IgM, hepatitis C antibody), antimitochondrial antibody (primary biliary cirrhosis), ANA, ceruloplasmin, urine copper (Wilson's disease), alpha-1-antitrypsin deficiency, drug screen, serum iron, TIBC, ferritin (hemochromatosis), liver biopsy.

Differential Diagnosis of Jaundice

Extrahepatic: Biliary tract disease (gallstone, stricture, cancer), infections (parasites, HIV, CMV, microsporidia); pancreatitis, pancreatic cancer.

Intrahepatic: Viral hepatitis, medication-related, acute fatty liver of pregnancy, alcoholic hepatitis, cirrhosis, primary biliary cirrhosis, autoimmune hepatitis, Wilson's disease, right heart failure, total parenteral nutrition; Dubin Johnson syndrome, Rotor's syndrome (direct hyperbilirubinemia); Gilbert's syndrome, Crigler-Niger syndrome (indirect); sclerosing cholangitis, sarcoidosis, amyloidosis, tumor.

Cirrhosis

History of the Present Illness: Jaundice, anorexia, nausea, fever; abdominal distension, abdominal pain, increased abdominal girth (ascites); vomiting, diarrhea, fatigue. Somnolence, confusion (encephalopathy); alcohol use. Viral hepatitis, blood transfusion, IV drug use.

Precipitating Factors of Encephalopathy: Gastrointestinal bleeding, high protein intake, constipation, azotemia, CNS depressants.

Physical Examination

General Appearance: Muscle wasting, fetor hepaticas (malodorous breath). Signs of dehydration. Note whether the patient looks "ill," well, or malnourished.

Vital Signs: Pulse, BP, temperature, respiratory rate.

Skin: Jaundice, spider angiomas (stellate, erythematous arterioles), palmar erythema; bronze skin discoloration (hemochromatosis), purpura, loss of body hair.

HEENT: Kayser-Fleischer rings (bronze corneal pigmentation, Wilson's disease), jugular venous distention (fluid overload). Parotid enlargement, sclera icterus, gingival hemorrhage (thrombocytopenia).

Chest: Bibasilar crackles, gynecomastia.

Abdomen: Bulging flanks, tenderness, rebound (peritonitis); fluid wave, shifting dullness, "puddle sign" (examiner flicks over lower abdomen while auscultating for dullness). Courvoisier's sign (palpable nontender gallbladder with jaundice; pancreatic malignancy); atrophic liver; liver margin texture (blunt, irregular, firm), splenomegaly. Umbilical or groin hernias (ascites).

Genitourinary: Scrotal edema, testicular atrophy.

Extremities: Lower extremity edema.

Neuro: Confusion, asterixis (jerking movement of hand with wrist hyperextended; hepatic encephalopathy).

Rectal: Occult blood, hemorrhoids.

Stigmata of Liver Disease: Spider angiomas (stellate red arterioles), jaundice, bronze discoloration (hemochromatosis), dilated periumbilical collateral veins (Caput medusae), ecchymoses, umbilical eversion, venous hum and thrill at umbilicus (Cruveilhier-Baumgarten syndrome); palmar erythema, Dupuytren's contracture (fibrotic palmar ridge to ring finger). Lacrimal and parotid gland enlargement, testicular atrophy, gynecomastia, ascites, encephalopathy, edema.

Labs: CBC, electrolytes, LFTs, albumin, INR/PTT, liver function tests, bilirubin, UA. Hepatitis serologies, antimitochondrial, antibody (primary, biliary cirrhosis), ANA, anti-Smith antibody, ceruloplasmin, urine copper (Wilson's disease), alpha-1-antitrypsin, serum iron, TIBC, ferritin (hemochromatosis).

Abdominal x-ray: Hepatic angle sign (loss of lower margin of right lateral liver angle), separation or centralization of bowel loops, generalized abdominal haziness (ascites). Ultrasound, paracentesis.

Differential Diagnosis of Cirrhosis: Alcoholic liver disease, viral hepatitis (B, C, D), hemochromatosis, primary biliary cirrhosis, autoimmune hepatitis, inborn error of metabolism (Crigler Najjar syndrome; Wilson's disease, alpha-1-antitrypsin deficiency), heart failure, venous outflow obstruction (Budd-Chiari, portal vein thrombus).

Evaluation of Ascites Fluid

Etiology	Appearance	Protein	Serum/fluid albumen ratio	RBC	WBC	Other
Cirrhosis	Straw	<3 g/dL	>1.1	low	<250 cells/mm^3	
Spontaneous Bacterial Peritonitis	Cloudy	<3	>1.1	low	>250 polys	Bacteria on gram stain and culture
Secondary Bacterial Peritonitis	Purulent	>3	<1.1	low	>10000	Bacteria on gram stain and culture
Neoplasm	Straw/bloody	>3	varies	high	>1000 lymphs	Malignant cells on cytology; triglycerides
Tuberculosis	Clear	>3	<1.1	low-high	>1000 lymphs	Acid fast bacilli
Heart Failure	Straw	>3	>1.1	low	<1000	
Pancreatitis	Turbid	>3	<1.1	varies	varies	Elevated amylase, lipase

Pancreatitis

History of the Present Illness: Constant, dull, boring, mid-epigastric or left upper quadrant pain; radiation to the mid-back; exacerbated by supine position, relieved by sitting with knees drawn up; nausea, vomiting, low-grade fever, rigors, jaundice; anorexia, dyspnea; elevated amylase.

Precipitating Factors: Alcohol, gallstones, trauma, postoperative, retrograde cholangiopancreatography, trauma, hypertriglyceridemia, hypercalcemia, renal failure, Coxsackie virus or mumps infection, mycoplasma infection. Lupus, vasculitis, penetration of peptic ulcer, scorpion stings, tumor.

Medications Associated with Pancreatitis: Sulfonamides, thiazides, dideoxyinosine (DDI), furosemide, tetracycline, estrogens, azathioprine, valproate, pentamidine.

Physical Examination

General Appearance: Signs of volume depletion, tachypnea. Septic appearance. Note whether the patient looks "ill," well, or malnourished.

Vital Signs: Temperature (low-grade fever), pulse (tachycardia), BP (hypotension), respirations (tachypnea).

Chest: Crackles, left lower lobe dullness (pleural effusion).

HEENT: Scleral icterus, Chvostek's sign (taping cheek results in facial spasm, hypocalcemia).

Skin: Jaundice, subcutaneous fat necrosis (erythematous skin nodules on legs and ankles); palpable purpura (polyarteritis nodosum).

Abdomen: Epigastric tenderness, distension; rigidity, rebound, guarding, hypoactive bowel sounds; upper abdominal mass; Cullen's sign (periumbilical bluish discoloration from hemoperitoneum), Grey-Turner's sign (bluish flank discoloration; retroperitoneal hemorrhage).

Extremities: Peripheral edema, anasarca.

Labs: Amylase, lipase, calcium, WBC, triglycerides, glucose, AST, LDL, UA.

Abdomen X-Rays: Ileus, pancreatic calcifications, obscure psoas margins, displaced or atonic stomach. Colon cutoff sign (spasm of splenic flexure with no distal colonic gas), diffuse ground-glass appearance (ascites).

Chest x-ray: Left plural effusion.

Ultrasound: Gallstones, pancreatic edema or enlargement.

CT scan with oral contrast: Pancreatic phlegmon, pseudocyst, abscess.

Ranson's Criteria of Pancreatitis Severity.

Early criteria: Age >55; WBC >16,000; glucose >200; LDH >350 IU/L; AST >250.

During initial 48 hours: Hematocrit decrease >10%; BUN increase >5; arterial pO2 <60 mmHg; base deficit >4 mEq/L; calcium <8; estimated fluid sequestration >6 L.

Differential Diagnosis of Midepigastric Pain: Pancreatitis, peptic ulcer, cholecystitis, hepatitis, bowel obstruction, mesenteric ischemia, renal colic, aortic dissection, pneumonia, myocardial ischemia.

Factors Associated with Pancreatitis: Alcoholic pancreatitis, gallstone pancreatitis, penetrating peptic ulcer, trauma, medications, hyperlipidemia, hypercalcemia, viral infections, pancreatic divisum, familial pancreatitis, pancreatic malignancy, methyl alcohol, scorpion stings, endoscopic retrograde cholangiopancreatography, vasculitis.

Gastritis and Peptic Ulcer Disease

History of the Present Illness: Recurrent, dull, burning, epigastric pain; 1-3 hours after meals; relieved by or worsen by food; worse when supine or reclining; relieved by antacids; awakens patient at night or in early morning. May radiate to back; nausea, vomiting, weight loss, coffee ground hematemesis; melena. Alcohol, salicylates, nonsteroidal anti-inflammatory drugs.

History of previous examinations: Endoscopy upper GI series, surgery; history of previous ulcer disease and Helicobacter pylori (HP) therapy.

Physical Examination

General Appearance: Mild distress. Signs of dehydration, septic appearance. Note whether the patient looks "ill," well, or malnourished.

Vital Signs: Pulse (tachycardia), BP (orthostatic hypotension), respiratory rate, temperature.

Skin: Pallor, delayed capillary refill.

Abdomen: Mild to moderate epigastric tenderness; rebound, rigidity, guarding (perforated ulcer), bowel sounds.

Rectal: Occult blood.

Labs: CBC, electrolytes, BUN, amylase, lipase. Abdominal x-ray series, endoscopy.

Differential Diagnosis: Pancreatitis, gastritis, gastroenteritis, perforating ulcer, intestinal obstruction, mesenteric adenitis, mesenteric thrombosis, aortic aneurysm, gastroesophageal reflux disease, non-ulcer dyspepsia.

Mesenteric Ischemia and Infarction

History of the Present Illness: Sudden onset of severe, poorly localized, periumbilical pain; pain is postprandial and may be relieved by nitroglycerine; frequent episodes of bloody diarrhea, nausea, vomiting, food aversion, weight loss,.

Peripheral vascular disease, claudication, chest pain, angina, myocardial infarction, atrial fibrillation, hypertension, hypercholesterolemia, diabetes, heart failure.

Physical Examination

General Appearance: Lethargy, mild to moderate distress. Signs of dehydration, septic appearance. Note whether the patient looks "cachectic," ill, well, or malnourished.

Vitals: Pulse, BP (orthostatic hypotension), pulse (tachycardia), respiratory rate, temperature.

HEENT: Atherosclerotic retinopathy, "silver wire" arteries; carotid bruits (mesenteric ischemia).

Skin: Cold, clammy skin, pallor, delayed capillary refill.

Abdomen: Initially hyperactive, then absent bowel sounds; peritoneal signs rebound, tenderness, distention, guarding, rigidity (peritoneal signs), pulsatile masses (aortic aneurysm), abdominal bruit.

Pain is usually out of proportion to the physical findings may be the only presenting symptom.

Extremities: Weak peripheral pulses, femoral bruits; asymmetric pulses (atherosclerotic disease).

Rectal: Occult or gross blood.

Labs: CBC, electrolytes, leukocytosis, hyperamylasemia. Hemoconcentration, prerenal azotemia, metabolic acidosis.

Chest x-ray: Free air under diaphragm (perforated viscus). Abdominal x-ray: "thumb-printing" (edema of intestinal wall), portal vein gas. Bowel wall gas (colonic ischemia, nonocclusive); angiogram.

Differential Diagnosis. Peritonitis, acute appendicitis, acute cholecystitis, perforated viscus, peptic ulcer, gastroenteritis, pancreatitis, bowel obstruction, carcinoma, ruptured aortic aneurysm.

Intestinal Obstruction

History of the Present Illness: Vomiting (bilious, feculent, bloody), nausea, obstipation, distention, crampy abdominal pain. Initially crampy or colicky pain with exacerbations every 5-10 minutes. Pain becomes diffuse with fever. Hernias, previous abdominal surgery, use of opiates, anticholinergics, antipsychotics, gallstones; colon cancer; history of constipation, recent weight loss, recent weight loss.

Pain localizes to periumbilical region in small bowel obstruction and localizes to lower abdomen in large bowel obstruction.

Physical Examination

General Appearance: Severe distress, signs of dehydration, septic appearance. Note whether the patient looks "ill," well, or malnourished.

Vital Signs: BP (hypotension), pulse (tachycardia), respiratory rate, temperature (fever).

Skin: Cold, clammy skin, pallor.

Abdomen: Hernias (incisional, inguinal, femoral, umbilical), scars (intraabdominal adhesions).

Bowel Sounds: High pitch rushes and tinkles coinciding with cramping (early) or absent bowel sounds (late).

Tenderness, rebound, rigidity, tender mass, distention, bruits.

Rectal: Gross blood, masses.

Labs: Leucocytosis, elevated BUN and creatinine, electrolytes; hypokalemic metabolic alkalosis due to vomiting, hyperamylasemia.

Abdominal x-rays: Dilated loops of small or large bowel, air-fluid levels, ladder pattern of dilated loops of bowel in the mid-abdomen. Colonic distention with haustral markings.

Causes of Small Bowel Obstruction: Adhesions (previous surgery), hernias, strictures from inflammatory processes; superior mesenteric artery syndrome, gallstone ileus. Ischemia, small bowel tumors, metastatic cancer.

Causes of Large Bowel Obstruction: Colon cancer, volvulus, diverticulitis, adynamic ileus, mesenteric ischemia, Ogilvie's syndrome (chronic pseudo-obstruction); narcotic ileus. Inflammatory bowel disease with stricture.

Differential Diagnosis: Myocardial infarction, cholecystitis, peptic ulcer, gastritis, gastroenteritis, peritonitis, sickle crisis, cancer, pancreatitis, renal colic.

Gynecologic Disorders

Amenorrhea

History of the Present Illness: Primary amenorrhea (absence of menses by age 16) or secondary amenorrhea (cessation of menses in a female with previously normal menstruation). Age of menarche, last menstrual period. Menstrual pattern, timing of breast and pubic hair development, sexual activity, possibility of pregnancy, pregnancy testing.

Life style changes, dieting and excessive exercise, medications (contraceptives) or drugs (marijuana), psychologic stress.

Hot flushes and night sweats (hypoestrogenism), galactorrhea (prolactinoma).

History of dilation and curettage, postpartum infection (Asherman's syndrome) or hemorrhage (Sheehan's syndrome), obesity, weight gain or loss, headaches, visual disturbances, thyroid symptoms; symptoms of pregnancy (nausea, breast tenderness), phenothiazines, antidepressants. Prior pregnancies.

Assess diet, medications or drugs.

Previous radiation therapy, chemotherapy.

Physical Examination

General Appearance: Secondary sexual characteristics, body habitus, obesity, signs of hyperthyroidism (tremor) or hypothyroidism (non-pitting edema, bradycardia, cool dry skin, hypothermia, brittle hair). Note whether the patient looks "ill," well, or malnourished.

HEENT: Acne, hirsutism, temporal balding, deepening of the voice (hyperandrogenism), visual field defects, thyroid enlargement or nodules.

Chest: Galactorrhea, breast development, breast atrophy.

Abdomen: Abdominal striae (Cushing's syndrome).

Gyn: Pubic hair distribution. Inguinal or labial masses, clitoromegaly, imperforate hymen, vaginal septum, vaginal atrophy, uterine enlargement, ovarian cysts or tumors.

Neuro: Focal motor deficits.

Labs: Pregnancy test, prolactin, TSH, free T_4. Progesterone-estrogen challenge testing.

Differential Diagnosis of Amenorrhea	
Pregnancy	**Outflow tract-related**
Hormonal contraception	Imperforate hymen
Hypothalamic-related	Transverse vaginal septum
Chronic or systemic illness	Agenesis of the vagina, cervix, uterus
Stress	Uterine synechiae
Athletics	**Androgen excess**
Eating disorder	Polycystic ovarian syndrome
Obesity	Adrenal tumor
Drugs	Adrenal hyperplasia (classic and
Tumor	nonclassic)
Pituitary-related	Ovarian tumor
Hypopituitarism	**Other endocrine causes**
Tumor	Thyroid disease
Infiltration	Cushing syndrome
Infarction	
Ovarian-related	
Dysgenesis	
Agenesis	
Ovarian failure	

Abnormal Uterine Bleeding

History of the Present Illness: Last menstrual period, age of menarche; regularity, duration and frequency of menses; amount of bleeding, number of pads per day; passing of clots; postcoital or intermenstrual bleeding; abdominal pain, fever, lightheadedness, sexual activity, possibility of pregnancy, birth control method, hormonal contraception.

Psychologic stress, weight changes, exercise. Changes in hair or skin texture or distribution

Molimina symptoms (premenstrual breast tenderness, bloating, dysmenorrhea). Obstetrical history.

Thyroid, renal, or hepatic diseases, coagulopathies. Adenomyosis, endometriosis, fibroids. Dental bleeding, endometrial biopsies.

Family history of coagulopathies, endocrine disorders.

Physical Examination

General Appearance: Assess rate of bleeding. Pallor, obesity, hirsutism, petechiae, skin and hair changes; fine thinning hair (hypothyroidism). Note whether the patient looks "ill," well, or malnourished, thyroid enlargement, galactorrhea.

Vital Signs: Assess hemodynamic stability, tachycardia, hypotension, orthostatic vitals; signs of shock.

Gyn: Cervical motion tenderness, adnexal tenderness, uterine size, cervical lesions. Cervical lesions should be biopsied.

Labs: CBC, platelets; serum pregnancy test; gonococcal culture, Chlamydia test, endometrial sampling. INR/PTT, bleeding time, type and screen.

Differential Diagnosis

Pregnancy-related. Ectopic pregnancy, abortion

Hormonal contraception

Hypothalamic-related. Chronic or systemic illness, stress, excessive exercise, eating disorders, obesity, drugs

Pituitary-related. Prolactinoma

Outflow tract-related. Trauma, foreign body, vaginal tumor, cervical carcinoma, endometrial polyp, uterine myoma, uterine carcinoma, intrauterine device

Androgen excess. Polycystic ovarian syndrome, adrenal tumor, ovarian tumor, adrenal hyperplasia (classic and nonclassic)

Other endocrine causes. Thyroid disease, adrenal disease

Hematologic-related. Thrombocytopenia, abnormalities of clotting factors, abnormalities of platelet function, anticoagulant medications

Infectious causes. Pelvic inflammatory disease, cervicitis

Pelvic Pain and Ectopic Pregnancy

History of the Present Illness: Positive pregnancy test, missed menstrual period, pelvic or abdominal pain (bilateral or unilateral), symptoms of pregnancy; abnormal vaginal bleeding (quantify). Menstrual interval, duration, age of menarche, obstetrical history.

Characteristics of pelvic pain; onset, duration; palliative or aggravating factors, shoulder pain. Rupture of ectopic pregnancy usually occurs 6-12 weeks after last menstrual period.

Associated Symptoms: Fever, vaginal discharge. Urinary or gastrointestinal symptoms, fever, abnormal bleeding, or vaginal discharge.

Past Medical History: Surgical history, gynecologic history, sexually transmitted diseases, Chlamydia, gonorrhea, infertility.

Method of Contraception: Oral contraceptives or barrier method, intrauterine device (IUD). Current sexual activity and practices.

Risk Factors for Ectopic Pregnancy: Prior pelvic infection, endometriosis, prior ectopic pregnancy, pelvic tumor, intrauterine device, pelvic/tubal surgery, infertility, diethylstilbestrol exposure in utero.

Physical Examination

General Appearance: Moderate to severe distress. Signs of dehydration, septic appearance. Note whether the patient looks "ill," well, or distressed.

Vital Signs: BP (orthostatic hypotension), pulse (tachycardia), respiratory rate, temperature (low fever).

Skin: Cold clammy skin, pallor, delayed capillary refill.

Abdomen: Cullen's sign (periumbilical darkening, intraabdominal bleeding), local then generalized tenderness, tenderness, rebound (peritoneal signs).

Pelvic: Cervical discharge, cervical motion tenderness; Chadwick's sign (cervical cyanosis; pregnancy); Hegar's sign (softening of uterine isthmus; pregnancy); enlarged uterus; tender adnexal mass or cul-de-sac fullness.

Labs: Quantitative beta-HCG, transvaginal ultrasound. Type and hold, Rh, CBC, UA with micro; GC, chlamydia culture. Laparoscopy.

Differential Diagnosis of Pelvic Pain

Pregnancy-Related Causes. Ectopic pregnancy, abortion (spontaneous, threatened, or incomplete), intrauterine pregnancy with corpus luteum bleeding.

Gynecologic Disorders. Pelvic inflammatory disease, endometriosis, ovarian cyst hemorrhage or rupture, adnexal torsion, Mittelschmerz, uterine leiomyoma torsion, primary dysmenorrhea, tumor.

Non-reproductive Tract Causes

Gastrointestinal. Appendicitis, inflammatory bowel disease, mesenteric adenitis, irritable bowel syndrome, diverticulitis.

Urinary Tract. Urinary tract infection, renal calculus.

Neurologic Disorders

Headache

History of the Present Illness: Quality of pain (dull, band-like, sharp, throbbing), location (retro-orbital, temporal, suboccipital, bilateral or unilateral), time course of typical headache episode; onset (gradual or sudden); exacerbating or relieving factors; time of day, effect of supine posture.

Age at onset of headaches; change in severity, frequency; awakening from sleep; analgesic or codeine use; family history of migraine. "The worst headache ever" (subarachnoid hemorrhage).

Aura or Prodrome: Visual scotomata, blurred vision; nausea, vomiting, sensory disturbances.

Associated Symptoms: Numbness, weakness, diplopia, photophobia, fever, nasal discharge (sinusitis); neck stiffness (meningitis); eye pain or redness (glaucoma); ataxia, dysarthria, transient blindness. Lacrimation, flushing, intermittent periodicity of headaches (cluster headaches).

Aggravating or Relieving Factors: Relief by analgesics or sleep. Exacerbation by foods (chocolate, alcohol, wine, cheese), emotional upset, menses; hypertension, trauma; lack of or excess sleep; exacerbation by fatigue, exertion, monosodium glutamate, nitrates.

Drugs: Nitrates, phenothiazines, sedatives, theophylline, sympathomimetics, estrogen, corticosteroids, excessive ergotamine, cold remedies, eye drops, diet pills, cocaine.

Symptoms of Depression: Sleep disturbance, decreased energy, loss of interest in usually pleasurable activities, poor concentration, depressed mood. Weight loss, decreased appetite.

Physical Examination

General Appearance: Note whether the patient looks "ill" or well.

Vital Signs: BP (hypertension), pulse, temperature (fever), respiratory rate.

HEENT: Cranial or temporal tenderness (temporal arteritis), asymmetric pupil reactivity; papilledema, extraocular movements, visual field deficits. Conjunctival injection, lacrimation, rhinorrhea (cluster headache).

Temporomandibular joint tenderness (TMJ syndrome); temporal or ocular bruits (arteriovenous malformation); sinus tenderness (sinusitis).

Dental infection, tooth tenderness to percussion (abscess); paraspinal muscle tenderness.

Neck: Neck rigidity.

Skin: Café au lait spots (neurofibromatosis), facial angiofibromas (adenoma sebaceum).

Neuro: Cranial nerve palsies (intracranial tumor); auditory acuity, focal weakness (intracranial tumor), sensory deficits, deep tendon reflexes, ataxia.

Labs: Electrolytes, ESR, MRI scan, lumbar puncture. CBC with differential, INR/PTT.

Indications for MRI scan: Focal neurologic signs, papilledema, decreased visual acuity, increased frequency or severity of headache, excruciating or paroxysmal headache, awakening from sleep, persistent vomiting, head trauma with focal neurologic signs or lethargy.

Differential Diagnosis: Migraine, tension headache; systemic infection, subarachnoid hemorrhage, sinusitis, arteriovenous malformation, hypertensive encephalopathy, temporal arteritis, meningitis, encephalitis, post concussion syndrome, intracranial tumor, venous sinus thrombosis, benign intracranial hypertension (pseudotumor cerebri), subdural hematoma, trigeminal neuralgia, post-herpetic neuralgia, glaucoma, analgesic overuse, psychogenic headache.

Characteristics of Migraine: Childhood to early adult onset; usually a family history; aura of scotomas or scintillations, unilateral pulsating or throbbing pain; nausea, vomiting. Lasts 2-6 hours; relief with sleep.

Characteristics of Tension Headache: Bilateral, generalized, bitemporal or suboccipital. Band-like pressure; throbbing pain, occurs late in day; related to stress. Onset in adolescence or young adult. Lasts hours and is usually relieved by simple analgesics.

Characteristics of Cluster Headache: Unilateral, retro-orbital searing pain. Lacrimation, nasal and conjunctival congestion. Young males; lasts 20-60 min. Occurs several times each day over several weeks, followed by pain-free periods.

Dizziness and Vertigo

History of the Present Illness: Sensation of spinning or movement of surroundings, light headedness, nausea, vomiting, tinnitus. Rate of onset and intensity of vertigo. Aggravation by change in position, turning of head, changing from supine to standing, coughing.

Hyperventilation, postural unsteadiness. Recent change in eyeglasses. Headache, hearing loss, head trauma.

Associated Symptoms: Recent upper respiratory infection, diplopia, paresthesias, syncope; hypertension, diabetes, history of stroke, transient ischemic attack, anemia, cardiovascular disease.

Drugs Associated with Vertigo: Antihypertensives, aspirin, alcohol, sedatives, diuretics, phenytoin, gentamicin, furosemide.

Physical Examination

General Appearance: Effect of hyperventilation on symptoms. Effect of Valsalva maneuver on symptoms. Note whether the patient looks "ill" or well.

Vital Signs: Pulse, BP (supine and upright, postural hypotension), respiratory rate, temperature.

HEENT: Nystagmus, visual acuity, visual field deficits, papilledema; facial weakness. Tympanic membrane inflammation (otitis media), cerumen. Effect of head turning or of placing the patient recumbent with head extended over edge of bed; Rinne's test (air/bone conduction); Weber test (lateralization of sound).

Heart: Rhythm, murmurs.

Neuro: Cranial nerves 2-12, sensory deficits, ataxia, weakness. Romberg test, coordination (finger to nose test), tandem gait.

Rectal: Occult blood.

Labs: CBC, electrolytes, MRI scan.

Differential Diagnosis

Drugs Associated with Vertigo: Aminoglycosides, loop diuretics, aspirin, caffeine, alcohol, phenytoin, psychotropics (lithium, haloperidol), benzodiazepines.

Peripheral Causes of Vertigo: Acute labyrinthitis/neuronitis, benign positional vertigo, Meniere's disease (vertigo, tinnitus, deafness), otitis media, acoustic neuroma, cerebellopontine angle tumor, cholesteatoma (chronic middle ear effusion), impacted cerumen.

Central Causes of Vertigo: Vertebrobasilar insufficiency, brain stem or cerebellar infarctions, tumors, encephalitis, meningitis, brain stem or cerebellar contusion, Parkinson's disease, multiple sclerosis.

Other Disorders Associated with Vertigo: Motion sickness, presyncope, syndrome of multiple sensory deficits (peripheral neuropathies, visual impairment, orthopedic problems), altered visual input (new eyeglasses), orthostatic hypotension.

Delirium, Coma and Confusion

History of the Present Illness: Level of consciousness, obtundation (awake but not alert), stupor (unconscious but awakable with vigorous stimulation), coma (cannot be awakened). Confusion, hallucination, formification (sensation that insects are crawling under skin); delirium, tremor, poor concentration, agitation.

Activity and symptoms prior to onset. Use of insulin, oral hypoglycemics, narcotics, alcohol, drugs, antipsychotics, anticholinergics, anticoagulants; history of trauma, suicide attempts or depression, epilepsy (post-ictal state).

Fever, headache; history of dementia, stroke, transient ischemic attacks, hypertension; renal, liver or cardiac disease.

Physical Examination

General Appearance: Signs of dehydration; septic appearance. Note whether the patient looks "ill," well, or malnourished.

Vital Signs: BP (hypertensive encephalopathy), pulse, temperature (fever), respiratory rate.

HEENT: Skull palpation for tenderness, lacerations. Pupil size and reactivity; extraocular movements, corneal reflexes. Papilledema, hemorrhages, flame lesions; facial asymmetry, ptosis, weakness. Battle's sign (ecchymosis over mastoid process), raccoon sign (periorbital ecchymosis, skull fracture), hemotympanum (basal skull fracture). Tongue or cheek lacerations (post-ictal state). Atrophic tongue (B12 deficiency).

Neck: Neck rigidity, carotid bruits.

Chest: Breathing pattern (Cheyne-Stokes hyperventilation); crackles, wheezes.

Heart: Rhythm, murmurs.

Abdomen: Hepatomegaly, splenomegaly, masses, ascites, tenderness, distention, dilated superficial veins (liver failure).

Extremities: Needle track marks (drug overdose), tatoos.

Skin: Cyanosis, jaundice, spider angiomata, palmar erythema (hepatic encephalopathy); capillary refill, petechia, splinter hemorrhages. Injection site fat atrophy (diabetes).

Neuro: Concentration (subtraction of serial 7s, delirium), strength, cranial nerves 2-12, mini-mental status exam; orientation to person, place, time, recent events; coordination, Babinski's sign, primitive reflexes (snout, suck, glabella, palmomental grasp). Tremor (Parkinson's disease, delirium tremens), incoherent speech, lethargy, somnolence.

Glasgow Coma Scale

Best Verbal Response: None - 1; incomprehensible sounds or cries - 2; appropriate words or vocal sounds - 3; confused speech or words - 4; oriented speech - 5.

Best Eye Opening Response: No eye opening - 1; eyes open to pain - 2; eyes open to speech - 3; eyes open spontaneously - 4.

Best Motor Response: None - 1; abnormal extension to pain - 2; abnormal flexion to pain - 3; withdraws to pain - 4; localizes to pain - 5; obeys commands - 6.

Total Score: 3-15

Special Neurologic Signs

Decortication: Painful stimuli causes flexion of arms, wrist and fingers with leg extension; indicates damage to contralateral hemisphere above midbrain.

Decerebration: Painful stimuli causes extension of legs and arms; wrists and fingers flex; indicates midbrain and pons functioning.

Oculocephalic Reflex (Doll's eyes maneuver): Eye movements in response to lateral rotation of head; no eye movements or loose movements occur with bihemispheric (diencephalon) lesions.

Oculovestibular Reflex (Cold caloric maneuver): Raise head 60 degrees and irrigate ear with cold water; causes tonic deviation of eyes to irrigated ear if intact brain stem; if the patient is conscious, nystagmus and vertigo will occur.

Labs: Glucose, electrolytes, calcium, BUN, creatinine, ABG. CT/MRI, ammonia, alcohol, liver function tests, urine toxicology screen, B-12, folate levels. LP if no signs of elevated intracranial pressure and suspicion of meningitis.

Differential Diagnosis of Delirium: Electrolyte imbalance, hyperglycemia, hypoglycemia (insulin overdose), alcohol or drug withdraw or intoxication, hypoxia, meningitis, encephalitis, systemic infection, stroke, intracranial hemorrhage, postictal state, exacerbation of dementia; narcotic or anticholinergic overdose; steroid withdrawal, hepatic encephalopathy; psychotic states, dehydration, hypertensive encephalopathy, head trauma, subdural hematoma, uremia, vitamin B12 or folate deficiency, hypothyroidism, ketoacidosis, factitious coma.

Weakness and Ischemic Stroke

History of the Present Illness: Rate and pattern of onset of weakness (gradual, sudden); time of onset and time course to maximum deficit; anatomic location of deficit; activity prior to onset (Valsalva, exertion, neck movement, sleeping); improvement or progression of symptoms; headache prior to event, nausea, vomiting, loss of consciousness; visual aura, vertigo, seizure.

Confusion, dysarthria, incontinence of stool or urine, dysphagia, palpitations; prior transient ischemic attacks (neurologic deficit lasting less than 24 hours) or strokes; past transient monocular blindness (Amaurosis fugax), tongue biting, tonic-clonic movements, head trauma.

Past Medical History: Hypertension, diabetes, coronary disease, endocarditis, hyperlipidemia, IV drug abuse, cocaine use, heart failure, valvular disease, arrhythmias (atrial fibrillation), claudication, anticoagulants, alcohol, antihypertensives, cigarette smoking.

Past testing: CT scans, carotid Doppler studies, echocardiograms.

Family history: Stroke, hyperlipidemia, cardiac disease.

Physical Examination

General Appearance: Level of consciousness, lethargy. Note whether the patient looks "ill" or well.

Vital Signs: BP, Pulse (bradycardia), temperature, respiratory rate. Cushing's response (bradycardia, hypertension, abnormal respirations).

HEENT: Signs of head trauma, pupil size and reactivity, extraocular movements. Fundi: hypertensive retinopathy, Roth spots (flame shaped lesions, endocarditis), retinal hemorrhages (subarachnoid hemorrhage), papilledema; facial asymmetry or weakness. Tongue lacerations.

Neck: Neck rigidity, carotid bruits.

Chest: Breathing pattern, Cheyne Stokes respiration (periodic breathing with periods of apnea, elevated intracranial pressure).

Heart: Irregular, irregular rhythm (atrial fibrillation), S3 (heart failure), murmurs (mitral stenosis, cardiogenic emboli).

Abdomen: Aortic pulsations, renal bruits (atherosclerotic disease).

Extremities: Unequal peripheral pulses, ecchymoses, trauma.

Skin: Petechia, splinter hemorrhages.

Neuro: Focal motor deficits, cranial nerves 2-12, gaze, ptosis, Babinski's sign (stroke sole of foot, and toes dorsiflex if pyramidal tract lesion). Clonus, primitive reflexes (snout, glabella, palmomental, grasp). Mini-mental status exam, memory concentration.

Signs of Increased Intracranial Pressure: Lethargy, headache, vomiting, meningismus, papilledema, focal neurologic deficits.

Signs of Cerebral Herniation: Obtundation, dilation of ipsilateral pupil, decerebrate posturing (extension of arms and legs in response to painful stimuli), ascending weakness. Cushing's response - bradycardia, hypertension, abnormal respirations.

Labs: CT scan: Bleeding, infarction, mass effect, midline shift. ECG, CBC.

Differential Diagnosis of Stroke: Infection (abscess, meningitis, encephalitis), subdural hematoma, brain tumor, metabolic imbalance (hypoglycemia, hypocalcemia), postictal paralysis (Todd's paralysis), delirium; conversion reaction; atypical migraine, basilar artery stenosis, transient ischemic attack.

Seizure

History of the Present Illness: Time of onset of seizure, duration of seizure, tonic-clonic movements, description of seizure. Past seizures, noncompliance with anticonvulsant medication (recent blood level). Aura (irritability, behavioral change, lethargy), pallor, incontinence of urine or feces, vomiting, post-ictal weakness or paralysis.

Prodrome (visual changes, paresthesias), stroke, migraine headaches, fever, chills. Diabetes (hypoglycemia), family history of epilepsy.

Factors that May Precipitate Seizures: Fatigue, sleep deprivation, infection, hyperventilation, head trauma, alcohol or drug withdrawal, cocaine intoxication; meningitis, high fever, uremia, hypoglycemia, theophylline toxicity, stroke.

Past testing: EEG's, CT scans.

Physical Examination

General Appearance: Post-ictal lethargy. Note whether the patient looks "ill" or well.

Vital Signs: BP (hypertension), pulse, respiratory rate, temperature (hyperpyrexia).

HEENT: Head trauma; pupil reactivity and equality, extraocular movements; papilledema, gum hyperplasia (phenytoin); tongue or buccal lacerations; carotid bruits, neck rigidity.

Chest: Rhonchi, wheeze (aspiration).

Heart: Rhythm, murmurs.

Extremities: Cyanosis, fractures, trauma.

Genitourinary/Rectal: Incontinence of urine or feces.

Skin: Café-au-lait spots, neurofibromas (Von Recklinghausen's disease), splinter hemorrhages (endocarditis). Unilateral port-wine facial nevus (Sturge-Weber syndrome); facial angiofibromas (adenoma sebaceum), hypopigmented ash leaf spots (tuberous sclerosis). Spider angiomas (hepatic encephalopathy).

Neuro: Dysarthria, sensory deficits, visual field deficits, focal weakness (Todd's paralysis), cranial nerves, Babinski's sign.

Labs: Glucose, electrolytes, calcium, liver function tests, CBC, urine toxicology, anticonvulsant levels, RPR/VDRL. EEG, MRI, lumbar puncture.

Differential Diagnosis: Epilepsy (complex partial seizure, generalized seizure), noncompliance with anticonvulsant medications, hypoglycemia, hyponatremia, hypocalcemia, hypomagnesemia, hypertensive encephalopathy, alcohol withdrawal, meningitis, encephalitis, brain tumor, stroke, vasculitis, pseudo-seizure.

Renal Disorders

Oliguria and Acute Renal Failure

History of the Present Illness: Oliguria (<20 mL/h, 400-500 mL urine/day); anuria (<100 mL urine/day); hemorrhage, heart failure, sepsis, infection, vomiting, nasogastric suction; diarrhea, fever, chills; measured fluid input and output by Foley catheter; prostate enlargement, kidney stones, anticholinergics.

Nephrotoxic drugs (aminoglycosides, amphotericin, NSAID's), dysuria, flank pain. Abdominal pain, hematuria, passing of tissue fragments, foamy urine (proteinuria). Administration of renally excreted medications.

Recent upper respiratory infection (post streptococcal glomerulonephritis), recent chemotherapy (tumor lysis syndrome).

Physical Examination

General Appearance: Signs of dehydration, septic appearance. Note whether the patient looks "ill" or well.

Vital Signs: BP (orthostatic vitals; an increase in heart rate by >15 mmHg and a fall in systolic pressure >15 mmHg, indicates significant volume depletion); pulse (tachycardia); temperature (fever), respiratory rate (tachypnea).

Skin: Decreased skin turgor over sternum (hypovolemia); skin temperature and color; delayed capillary refill; jaundice (hepatorenal syndrome).

HEENT: Oral mucous membrane moisture, ocular moisture, flat neck veins (volume depletion), venous distention (heart failure).

Chest: Crackles (heart failure).

Heart: S3 (volume overload).

Abdomen: Hepatomegaly, abdominojugular reflex (heart failure); costovertebral angle tenderness; distended bladder, nephromegaly (obstruction).

Pelvic: Pelvic masses, cystocele, urethrocele.

Rectal: Prostate hypertrophy; absent sphincter reflex, decreased sensation (atonic bladder due to vertebral disk herniation).

Extremities: Peripheral edema (heart failure).

Labs: Sodium, potassium, BUN, creatinine, uric acid. Urine and serum osmolality, UA, urine creatinine. Ultrasound of bladder and kidneys.

Fractional excretion of sodium (FE Na) =
$$\frac{UNa(mMol/L) \times SCr(mmol/L)}{SNa(mMol/L) \quad UCr(mMol/L)} \times 100$$

Renal Failure Index =
$$\frac{UNa \times 100}{U/PCr}$$

Clinical Findings in Pre-renal, Renal, Post-renal Failure			
	Prerenal	ARF	Postrenal
BUN/Creatinine ratio	>15:1	<15:1	varies
Urine sodium	<20 mMol/L	>20	varies
Urine osmolality	>500 mOsm/kg	<350	varies
Renal failure Index	<1	>1	varies
FE Na	<1%	>1%	varies
Urine/plasma creatinine	>40	>20	varies
Urine analyses	normal	cellular casts	RBCs, WBCs, bacteria

Differential Diagnosis of Acute Renal Failure
Prerenal Insult
A. Prerenal insult is the most common cause of acute renal failure, accounting for 70%.
B. It is usually caused by reduced renal perfusion pressure secondary to extracellular fluid volume loss (diarrhea, diuresis, GI hemorrhage), or secondary to extracellular fluid sequestration (pancreatitis, sepsis), inadequate cardiac output, renal vasoconstriction (sepsis, liver disease), or inadequate fluid intake or replacement.

Intrarenal Insult
A. Insult to the renal parenchyma (tubular necrosis) causes 20% of acute renal failure.
B. Prolonged hypoperfusion is the most common cause of tubular necrosis.
C. Nephrotoxins (radiographic contrast, aminoglycosides) are the second most common cause of tubular necrosis.
D. Pigmenturia induced renal injury can be caused by intravascular hemolysis or rhabdomyolysis.
E. Acute glomerulonephritis or acute inflammation of renal interstitium (acute interstitial nephritis) (usually from allergic reactions to beta-lactam antibiotics, sulfonamides, rifampin, NSAIDs, cimetidine, phenytoin, allopurinol, thiazides, furosemide, analgesics) are occasional causes of intrarenal kidney failure.

Postrenal Insult

    A. Postrenal damage results from obstruction of urine flow, and it is the least common cause of acute renal failure, accounting for 10%.

    B. Postrenal insult may be caused by extrarenal obstructive uropathy (prostate cancer, benign prostatic hypertrophy, renal calculi obstruction) or by intrarenal obstruction (amyloidosis, uric acid crystals, multiple myeloma, or acyclovir).

Chronic Renal Failure

History of the Present Illness: Oliguria, current and baseline creatinine, and BUN. Diabetes, hypertension; history of pyelonephritis, sepsis, heart failure, liver disease; peripheral edema, dark colored urine, rashes or purpura; medications (nonsteroidal anti-inflammatory drugs, aminoglycosides, contrast dyes). Hypovolemia secondary to diarrhea, hemorrhage, over-diuresis; glomerulonephritis, interstitial nephritis.

Past ultrasounds, flank pain, history of kidney stones, prostate disease, urethral obstruction. Anorexia, insomnia, fatigue, malaise, weight loss, bleeding diathesis, paresthesias, anemia.

Family history of polycystic kidney disease, hereditary glomerulonephritis.

Physical Examination

General Appearance: Evaluate intravascular volume status. Signs of fluid overload. Note whether the patient looks "ill," well, or malnourished.

Vital Signs: Postural blood pressure and pulse (tachycardia, hypertension), temperature (fever), respiratory rate.

Skin: Skin turgor, sallow yellow skin (urochromes), fine white powder (uremic frost), purpura, petechiae (coagulopathy). Jaundice, spider angiomas (hepatorenal syndrome).

HEENT: Neck vein distention (volume overload).

Chest: Crackles (rales).

Heart: S3 gallop (volume overload), cardiac friction rub (pericarditis), displacement of heart border, muffled heart sounds (effusion), arrhythmias (electrolyte imbalances).

Abdomen: Distended bladder, costovertebral angle or suprapubic tenderness, pelvic masses, ascites.

Rectal: Occult blood, prostate enlargement.

Neuro: Asterixis, myoclonus, sensory deficits.

Labs: BUN, creatinine, potassium (hyperkalemia), albumin, calcium, phosphorus, proteinuria.

Differential Diagnosis of Chronic Renal Failure: Hypertensive nephrosclerosis, diabetic nephrosclerosis, glomerulonephritis, polycystic kidney disease, tubulointerstitial renal disease, reflux nephropathy, analgesic nephropathy, chronic obstructive uropathy, amyloidosis, Lupus nephropathy.

Hematuria

History of the Present Illness: Frequency, dysuria, suprapubic pain, flank pain (renal colic), abdominal or perineal pain; fever. Recent exercise, menstruation; bleeding between voidings.

Foley catheterization, prior stone passage, tissue passage in urine, joint pain.

Color, timing, pattern of hematuria: Initial hematuria (anterior urethral lesion); terminal hematuria (bladder neck or prostate lesion); hematuria throughout voiding (bladder or upper urinary tract).

Recent sore throat, streptococcal skin infection (glomerulonephritis). Prior pyelonephritis, joint pain; occupational exposure to toxins.

Family History: Hematuria, renal disease, sickle cell, bleeding diathesis, deafness (Alport's syndrome), hypertension.

Medications Associated with Hematuria: Warfarin, aspirin, ibuprofen, naproxen, phenobarbital, allopurinol, phenytoin, cyclophosphamide.

Causes of Red Urine: Pyridium, phenytoin, ibuprofen, cascara laxatives, levodopa, methyldopa, quinine, rifampin, berries, flava beans, food coloring, rhubarb, beets, hemoglobinuria, myoglobinuria.

Physical Examination

General Appearance: Signs of dehydration. Note whether the patient looks "ill," well, or malnourished.

Vital Signs: BP (hypertension).

Skin: Rashes.

HEENT: Pharyngitis, carotid bruits.

Heart: Heart murmur; irregular, irregular (atrial fibrillation, renal emboli).

Abdomen: Tenderness, masses, costovertebral angle tenderness (renal calculus or pyelonephritis), abdominal bruits, nephromegaly, suprapubic tenderness.

Genitourinary: Urethral lesions, discharge, condyloma, foreign body, cervical malignancy; prostate tenderness, nodules, or enlargement (prostatitis, prostate cancer).

Extremities: Peripheral edema (nephrotic syndrome), arthritis, ecchymoses, petechiae, unequal peripheral pulses (aortic dissection).

Labs: UA with microscopic exam of urinary sediment, CBC, KUB, intravenous pyelogram, ultrasound. Streptozyme panel, ANA, INR/PTT.

Indicators of Significant Hematuria: (1) >3 RBC's per high-power field on 2 of 3 specimens; (2) >100 RBC's per HPF in 1 specimen; (3) gross hematuria

The patient should abstain from exercise for 48 hours prior to urine collection, and it should not be collected during menses.

Differential Diagnosis

   A. Medical Hematuria is caused by a glomerular lesion; plasma proteins filter into urine out of proportion to the amount of hematuria. It is characterized by glomerular RBCs that are distorted with crenated membranes and an uneven hemoglobin distribution and casts. Microscopic hematuria and a urine dipstick test of 2+ protein is more likely to have a medical cause.

   B. Urologic Hematuria is caused by a urologic lesion such as a urinary stone or carcinoma; it is characterized by minimal proteinuria, and protein appears in urine proportional to the amount of whole blood present. RBCs are disk shaped with an even hemoglobin distribution, and there is an absence of casts.

Nephrolithiasis

History of the Present Illness: Severe, colicky, intermittent, migrating, lower abdominal pain; flank pain, hematuria, fever, dysuria; prior history of renal stones. Pain is not associated with position; abdominal pain may radiate laterally around abdomen to groin, testicles or labia. History of low fluid intake, urinary tract infection, parenteral nutrition.

Excessive calcium administration, immobilization, furosemide, neurogenic bladder, chemotherapy; family history of kidney stones. Inflammatory bowel disease, ileal resection. Diet high in oxalate: Spinach, rhubarb, nuts, tea, cocoa. Excess vitamin C intake, hydrochlorothiazide, indinavir; unusual dietary habits.

Physical Examination

General Appearance: Signs of dehydration, septic appearance. Note whether the patient looks "ill," well, or malnourished.

Abdomen: Costovertebral angle tenderness, suprapubic tenderness; enlarged kidney. Pelvic examination for cervical motion tenderness, adnexal tenderness.

Labs: Serum calcium, phosphorus, bicarbonate, creatinine, uric acid. Urine cystine, UA microscopic (hematuria), urine culture, intravenous pyelogram.

Differential Diagnosis: Nephrolithiasis, cystitis, diverticulitis, appendicitis, salpingitis, torsion of hernia, ovarian torsion, ovarian cyst rupture or hemorrhage, bladder obstruction, prostatitis, prostate cancer, endometriosis, ectopic pregnancy, colonic obstruction, carcinoma (colon, prostrate, cervix, bladder).

Causes of Nephrolithiasis: Hypercalcemia, hyperuricosuria, hyperoxaluria, cystinuria, renal tubular acidosis, Proteus mirabilis urinary tract infection with staghorn calculi.

Hyperkalemia

History of the Present Illness: Serum potassium >5.5 mMol/L (repeat test to exclude lab error); muscle weakness, syncope, lightheadedness, palpitations, oliguria; excess intake of oral or intravenous potassium, salt substitutes, potassium sparing diuretics, angiotensin converting enzyme inhibitors; nonsteroidal anti-inflammatory drugs, beta blockers, heparin, digoxin toxicity cyclosporine, succinylcholine; muscle trauma, chemotherapy (tumor lysis syndrome).

History of renal disease, diabetes, adrenal insufficiency (Addison's syndrome). History of episodic paralysis precipitated by exercise (familial hyperkalemic periodic paralysis).

Physical Examination

General Appearance: Dehydration. Note whether the patient looks "ill," well, or malnourished.

Skin: Hyperpigmentation (Addison's disease), hematomas.

Abdomen: Suprapubic tenderness.

Neuro: Muscle weakness, abnormal deep tendon reflexes, cranial nerves 2-12.

Labs: Potassium, platelets, bicarbonate, chloride, anion gap, LDH, urine K, pH. Serum aldosterone, plasma renin activity.

ECG: Tall peaked, precordial T waves; diminished QT interval; widened QRS complex, prolonged PR interval, P wave flattening, AV block, ventricular arrhythmias, sine wave, asystole.

Differential Diagnosis

Inadequate Excretion: Renal failure, adrenal insufficiency (Addison's syndrome), potassium sparing diuretics (spironolactone), urinary tract obstruction, lupus, hypoaldosteronism, ACE inhibitors, NSAIDs, heparin.

Increased Potassium Production: Hemolysis, rhabdomyolysis, muscle crush injury, internal hemorrhage, drugs (succinylcholine, digoxin overdose, beta blockers), acidosis, hyperkalemic periodic paralysis, hyperosmolality.

Excess Intake of Potassium: Oral or IV potassium supplements, salt substitutes.

Pseudo-hyperkalemia: Hemolysis after collection of blood, use of excessively small needle, excessive shaking of sample, delayed transport of blood to lab, thrombocytosis, leukocytosis, prolonged tourniquet use.

Hypokalemia

History of the Present Illness: Potassium <3.5 mMol/L (repeat test to exclude lab error), hyperglycemia, diuretics, diarrhea, vomiting, laxative abuse; poor intake of potassium containing foods; corticosteroids, nephrotoxins, bicarbonate, beta agonists. Conn's syndrome (hyperaldosteronism).

Associated Symptoms: Muscle weakness, cramping pain, nausea, vomiting, constipation, palpitations, paresthesias, polyuria.

Precipitating Factors: Renal disease, stress (catecholamine release), vitamin B12 treatment; biliary drainage, enteric fistula; Kayexalate ingestion, dialysis, excessive licorice ingestion, chewing tobacco.

Physical Examination

General Appearance: Signs of dehydration. Note whether the patient looks "ill," well, or malnourished.

Vital Signs: BP, pulse, temperature, respiratory rate.

Heart: Rate and rhythm.

Abdomen: Hypoactive bowel sounds (ileus).

Neuro: Weakness, hypoactive tendon reflexes.

Labs: Serum potassium. 24 hour urine potassium >20 mEq/day indicates excessive urinary K loss. If <20 mEq/d, low K intake or nonurinary K loss is the cause. Electrolytes, BUN, creatinine, glucose, magnesium, CBC, plasma renin activity, aldosterone. Urine specific gravity.

ECG: Flattening and inversion of T-waves (II, V3), ST segment depression, U waves (II, V1, V2, V3); first or second degree block, QT interval prolongation, premature atrial or ventricular contractions, supraventricular tachycardia, ventricular tachycardia or fibrillation.

Differential Diagnosis of Hypokalemia

Cellular Redistribution of Potassium: Intracellular shift of potassium by insulin (exogenous or glucose load), beta2 agonist; thyrotoxic periodic paralysis; alkalosis-induced shift (metabolic or respiratory); familial periodic paralysis, vitamin B12 treatment, hypothermia; acute myeloid leukemia.

Nonrenal Potassium Loss:

Gastrointestinal Loss. Diarrhea, laxative abuse, villous adenoma, biliary drainage, enteric fistula, potassium binding resin ingestion

Non-gastrointestinal Loss. Sweating, low potassium ingestion, dialysis

Renal Potassium Loss:

Hypertensive High Renin States. Malignant hypertension, renal artery stenosis, renin-producing tumor.

Hypertensive Low Renin, High Aldosterone States. Primary hyperaldosteronism (adenoma or hyperplasia).

Hypertensive Low Renin, Low Aldosterone States. Congenital adrenal hyperplasia, Cushing's syndrome, exogenous mineralocorticoids (Florinef, licorice, chewing tobacco), Liddle's syndrome

Normotensive. Renal tubular acidosis (type I or II), metabolic alkalosis with a urine chloride <10 mEq/day is caused by vomiting; metabolic alkalosis with a urine chloride >10 mEq/day is caused by Bartter's syndrome, diuretics, magnesium depletion, normotensive hyperaldosteronism

Hyponatremia

History of the Present Illness: Serum sodium <135 mMol/L (repeat test to exclude lab error); decreased mental status, confusion, agitation, irritability, lethargy, anorexia, nausea, vomiting, headache, muscle weakness or tremor, cramps, seizures; decreased output of dark urine (dehydration); polydipsia (water intoxication); diuretics, diarrhea, steroid withdrawal.

Renal, CNS, or pulmonary disease (syndrome of inappropriate antidiuretic hormone); heart failure, cirrhosis; hypotonic IV fluids, psychotropic medications, chemotherapeutic agents, hypothyroidism, hyperlipidemia (pseudohyponatremia).

Physical Examination

General Appearance: Signs of dehydration. Note whether the patient looks "ill," well, or malnourished.

Vital Signs: BP, pulse (orthostatic vitals), temperature, respiratory rate.

Skin: Decreased skin turgor, delayed capillary refill; hyperpigmentation (Addison's disease), moon-face, truncal obesity (hypocortisolism with steroid withdrawal).

HEENT: Decreased ocular and oral moisture.

Chest: Cheyne-Stokes respirations, crackles.

Heart: Rhythm and rate. Premature ventricular contractions.

Abdomen: Ascites, tenderness.

Extremities: Edema.

Neuro: Confusion, irritability, motor weakness, ataxia, positive Babinski's sign, muscle twitches; hypoactive deep tendon reflexes, cranial nerve palsies.

Labs: Electrolytes, BUN, creatinine, cholesterol, triglycerides, glucose, protein, osmolality, albumin; urine sodium, urine osmolality, chest x-ray, ECG.

Differential Diagnosis of Hyponatremia Based on Urine Osmolality

    A. Low Urine Osmolality (50-180 mOsm/L). Primary excessive water intake (psychogenic water drinking).

    B. High Urine Osmolality (urine osmolality >serum osmolality)

        1. **High Urine Sodium (>40 mEq/L) and Volume Contracted.** Renal fluid loss (excessive diuretic use, salt-wasting nephropathy,

Addison's disease, osmotic diuresis).

2. **High Urine Sodium (>40 mEq/L) and Normal Volume.** Water retention caused by a drug (carbamazepine, cyclophosphamide), hypothyroidism, syndrome of inappropriate antidiuretic hormone secretion.

3. **Low Urine Sodium (<20 mEq/L) and Volume Contraction.** Extrarenal source of fluid loss (vomiting, burns).

4. **Low Urine Sodium (<20 mEq/L) and Volume-expanded, Edematous.** Heart failure, cirrhosis with ascites, nephrotic syndrome.

Hypernatremia

History of the Present Illness: Serum sodium >145 mEq/L (repeat test to exclude lab error). History of dehydration due to fever, vomiting, burns, heat exposure, diarrhea, elevated glucose, salt ingestion, administration of hypertonic fluids (sodium bicarbonate, sodium chloride), sweating, impaired access to water (elderly), adipsia (lack of thirst); head injury.

Altered mental status, lethargy, agitation, polyuria, anorexia, muscle twitching, renal disease. Recent fluid intake.

Drugs causing hypernatremia: Amphotericin, phenytoin, lithium, aminoglycosides.

Physical Examination

General Appearance: Lethargy, obtundation, stupor. Note whether the patient looks "ill," well, or malnourished.

Vital Signs: BP (orthostatic hypotension), pulse (tachycardia), temperature, respiratory rate; decreased urine output.

Skin: Decreased skin turgor ("doughy" consistency), delayed capillary refill, hyperpigmentation (Conn's syndrome), moon-face, truncal obesity, stria (hypoadrenal crisis, steroid withdrawal).

HEENT: Dry mucous membranes, flat neck veins, decreased eye turgor.

Neuro: Decreased muscle tone, ataxia, tremor, hyperreflexia; extensor plantar reflexes (Babinski's sign), spasticity.

Labs: Increased hematocrit; sodium, BUN, creatinine, urine and serum, osmolality. Spot urine sodium, creatinine.

Differential Diagnosis:

Hypernatremia with Hypovolemia

    A. **Extrarenal Loss of Water (urine sodium >20 mMol/L).** Vomiting, diarrhea, sweating, pancreatitis, respiratory water loss.

    B. **Renal loss of water (urine sodium <10 mMol/L).** Diuretics, hyperglycemia, renal failure.

Euvolemic Hypernatremia with Renal Water Losses. Diabetes insipidus (central or nephrogenic secretion of excessive antidiuretic hormone).

Hypernatremia with Hypervolemia (urine sodium >20 mMol/L): Hypertonic solutions of sodium chloride or sodium bicarbonate, hyperaldosteronism, Cushing's, syndrome, congenital adrenal hyperplasia.

Endocrinologic Disorders

Diabetic Ketoacidosis

History of the Present Illness: Initial glucose level, ketones, anion gap. Polyuria, polyphagia, polydipsia, fatigue, lethargy, nausea, vomiting, weight loss; noncompliance with insulin, hypoglycemic agents, or diet; blurred vision, physical stress, infection, dehydration, abdominal pain (appendicitis), dyspnea.

Cough, fever, chills, ear pain (otitis media), dysuria, frequency (urinary tract infection); back pain (pyelonephritis), chest pain; frequent Candida albicans or bacterial infections.

Factors that May Precipitate Diabetic Ketoacidosis. New onset of diabetes, noncompliance with insulin, infection, pancreatitis, myocardial infarction, stress, trauma, stroke, pregnancy.

Renal disease, prior ketoacidosis, sensory deficits in extremities (diabetic neuropathy), retinopathy, hypertension.

Physical Examination

General Appearance: Somnolence, Kussmaul respirations (deep sighing breathing). Signs of dehydration, toxic appearance. Note whether the patient looks "ill," well, or malnourished.

Vital Signs: BP (orthostatic hypotension), pulse (tachycardia), temperature (fever or hypothermia), respiratory rate (tachypnea).

Skin: Decreased skin turgor, delayed capillary refill; hyperpigmented atrophic macules on legs (shin spots); intertriginous candidiasis, erythrasma, localized fat atrophy (insulin injections).

HEENT: Diabetic retinopathy (neovascularization, hemorrhages, exudates); acetone breath odor (musty, apple odor), decreased visual acuity, low oral moisture (dehydration), tympanic membrane inflammation (otitis media); flat neck veins, neck rigidity.

Chest: Rales, rhonchi.

Abdomen: Hypoactive bowel sounds (ileus), abdominal tenderness, costovertebral angle tenderness (pyelonephritis), suprapubic tenderness (urinary tract infection).

Extremities: Decreased pulses (atherosclerotic disease), foot ulcers, cellulitis.

Neuro: Delirium, confusion, peripheral neuropathy (decreased proprioception and sensory deficits in feet), hypotonia, hyporeflexia.

Labs: Glucose, sodium, potassium, bicarbonate, chloride, BUN, creatinine, anion gap; triglycerides, phosphate, CBC, serum ketones; UA (proteinuria, ketones). Chest x-ray, ECG.

Differential Diagnosis

Ketosis-Causing Conditions. Alcoholic ketoacidosis or starvation.

Acidosis-Causing Conditions

Increased Anion Gap Acidoses. DKA, lactic acidosis, uremia, and salicylate or methanol poisoning.

Non-Anion Gap Acidoses. Renal or gastrointestinal bicarbonate losses due to diarrhea or renal tubular acidosis.

Hyperglycemia-Causing Conditions. Hyperosmolar nonketotic coma.

Diagnostic Criteria for DKA. Glucose ≥250, pH <7.3, bicarbonate <15, ketone positive >1:2 dilutions.

Hypothyroidism and Myxedema Coma

History of the Present Illness: Fatigue, cold intolerance, constipation, weight gain or inability to lose weight, muscle weakness; thyroid swelling or mass; dyspnea on exertion; mental slowing, dry hair and skin, deepening of voice; carpal tunnel syndrome, amenorrhea.

Past history of hyperthyroidism, thyroid testing, thyroid surgery or radioactive iodine treatment, antithyroid medication, lithium.

Somnolence, apathy, depression.

Myxedema madness: Agitation, disorientation, delusions, hallucinations, paranoia, restlessness, lethargy.

Factors Predisposing to Myxedema Coma. Cold exposure, infection, trauma, surgery, anesthesia, narcotics, phenothiazines, phenytoin, sedatives, propranolol, alcohol.

Physical Examination

General Appearance: Hypoactivity, confusion, somnolence, coarse, deep voice; dull, expressionless face. Signs of dehydration.

Vital Signs: Bradycardia, hypotension, hypothermia.

Skin: Cool, dry, pale, rough, doughy skin; thin, brittle dry nails with longitudinal ridges; yellowish skin without scleral icterus (carotenemia). Hyperkeratosis of elbows and knees.

HEENT: Thin, dry, brittle hair, alopecia; macroglossia (enlarged tongue), puffy face and eyelids; loss of lateral third of eyebrows, papilledema, thyroid surgery scar. Jugular venous distention (pericardial effusion).

Chest: Dullness to percussion (pleural effusion).

Heart: Muffled heart sounds (pericardial effusion); displacement of lateral heart border, bradycardia.

Abdomen: Hypoactive bowel sounds (ileus), myxedematous ascites.

Extremities: Diminished muscle strength and power. Myxedema: transient local swelling after tapping a muscle.

Neuro: Visual field deficits, cranial nerve palsies (pituitary tumor), hypoactive tendon reflexes with delayed return phase. Decreased mental status, stupor, ataxia; paresthesias, weakness, sensory impairment.

Labs: Thyroid stimulating hormone, CBC, electrolytes, hypercholesterolemia, hypertriglyceridemia, creatinine phosphokinase, LDH.

ECG: Bradycardia, low voltage QRS complexes; flattened or inverted T waves, prolonged Q-T interval.

Differential Diagnosis of Hypothyroidism	
Cause	Clues to Diagnosis
Autoimmune thyroiditis (Hashimoto's disease)	Family or personal history of auto-immune thyroiditis or goiter
Iatrogenic: Ablation, medication, surgery	History of thyroidectomy, irradia-tion with iodine 131, or thio-amide drug therapy
Diet (high levels of iodine)	Kelp consumption
Subacute thyroiditis (viral)	History of painful thyroid gland or neck pain
Postpartum thyroiditis	Symptoms of hyperthyroidism fol-lowed by hypothyroidism 6 months postpartum

Hyperthyroidism and Thyrotoxicosis

History of the Present Illness: Tremor, nervousness, hyperkinesis (restless-ness), fever, heat intolerance, palpitations, diaphoresis, irritability, insomnia; thyroid enlargement, masses, thyroid pain, amenorrhea.

Weight loss with increased appetite; dyspnea and fatigue after slight exertion; softening of the skin; fine, silky hair texture; proximal muscle weakness (especially thighs when climbing stairs), hyperdefecation.

Atrial fibrillation; diplopia, reduced visual acuity, eye discomfort or pain, lacrimation; recent upper respiratory infection. Previous thyroid function testing; family history of thyroid disease.

Factors Precipitating Thyroid Storm: Infection, surgery, diabetic ketoacidosis, pulmonary embolus, excess hormone medication, cerebral vascular accident, myocardial infarction, labor and delivery, iodine-131 or iodine therapy.

Physical Examination

General Appearance: Restless, anxious, hyperactive; delirium. Signs of dehydration.

Vital Signs: Widened pulse pressure (difference between systolic and diastolic pressure), hyperpyrexia (>104°F), tachycardia, hypertension.

Skin: Moist, warm, velvety skin, diaphoresis; palmar erythema, fine silky hair. Plummer's nails (distal onycholysis, separation of fingernail from nail bed), clubbing of fingers and toes (acropachy). Loss of subcutaneous fat and muscle mass.

HEENT: Exophthalmos (forward displacement of the eyeballs), proptosis, widened palpebral fissures; lid lag, infrequent blinking.

Ophthalmoplegia (restricted extraocular movements), chemosis (edema of conjunctiva), conjunctival injection, corneal ulcers; periorbital edema or ecchymoses; optic nerve atrophy, impaired visual acuity, difficulty with convergence. Painless, diffusely enlarged, thyroid without masses; thyroid thrill and bruit.

Heart: Irregular, irregular rhythm (atrial fibrillation), systolic murmur (mitral or tricuspid regurgitation, flow murmur), displacement of apical impulse. Accentuated first heart sound.

Extremities: Fine tremor; non-pitting pre-tibial edema (Grave's disease).

Neuro: Proximal muscle weakness, hyperreflexia (rapid return phase of deep tendon reflexes); rapid, pressured speech, anxiety.

Labs: Free T4, TSH, beta-HCG pregnancy test.

ECG: Sinus tachycardia, atrial fibrillation.

Differential Diagnosis: Grave's disease, toxic multinodular goiter, acute thyroiditis, thyrotoxicosis factitia (ingestion of thyroid hormone), trophoblastic tumor (molar pregnancy), TSH producing pituitary adenoma, postpartum thyroiditis, ectopic thyroid tissue (struma ovarii, functional follicular carcinoma), thyroid adenoma or carcinoma.

Hematologic and Rheumatologic Disorders

Deep Venous Thrombosis

History of the Present Illness: Sudden onset of unilateral calf pain, swelling, and redness; exacerbation of pain by walking and flexing of foot, dyspnea.

Risk Factors for Deep Venous Thrombosis

    A. **Venous stasis** risk factors include prolonged immobilization, stroke, myocardial infarction, heart failure, obesity, anesthesia, age >65 years old.

    B. **Endothelial injury** risk factors include surgery, trauma, central venous access catheters, pacemaker wires, previous thromboembolic event.

    C. **Hypercoagulable state** risk factors include malignant disease, high estrogen level (pregnancy, oral contraceptives).

    D. **Hematologic Disorders.** Polycythemia, leukocytosis, thrombocytosis, antithrombin III deficiency, protein C deficiency, protein S deficiency, antiphospholipid syndrome.

Past Medical History: Peptic ulcer, melena, surgery.

Physical Examination

General Appearance: Dyspnea, respiratory distress. Note whether the patient looks "ill," well, or malnourished.

Vital Signs: BP, pulse, respiratory rate (tachypnea if pulmonary embolus), temperature (low-grade fever).

Chest: Breast masses.

Abdomen: Distention, tenderness, masses.

Genitourinary/Rectal: Occult fecal blood, prostate masses, testicular or pelvic masses, inguinal lymphadenopathy.

Extremities: >2 cm difference in calf circumference, redness, cyanosis; mottling, tenderness; Homan's sign (tenderness with dorsiflexion of foot); warmth, dilated varicose veins.

Labs: Doppler studies, venogram; INR/PTT, CBC, electrolytes, BUN, creatinine; ECG, UA, chest x-ray.

Differential Diagnosis: Thrombophlebitis, ruptured Baker's cyst, lymphatic obstruction, cellulitis, muscle injury, hematoma, plantaris tendon rupture.

Connective Tissue Diseases

History of the Present Illness: Joint pain, fatigue, malaise, weight loss, fever, skin rashes; swelling of upper and lower extremities, morning joint stiffness, photosensitivity, muscle aches, weakness.

Hip and back pain, oral ulcers, renal disease; anemia, psychiatric illness, dysphagia, pleurisy, positional chest pain (pericarditis), Raynaud's syndrome (cyanosis of hands when exposed to cold); migraine headaches, stroke, depression, hypertension.

Drugs Associated with Lupus: Procainamide, isoniazid, hydralazine, methyldopa (Aldomet).

Physical Examination

General Appearance: Note whether the patient looks "ill," well, or malnourished.

Vital Signs: Hypertension

Skin: Skin fibrosis (thickening, scleroderma), telangiectasias, discoid lesions (erythematous plaques), purpura, skin ulcers, rheumatoid nodules, livedo reticularis.

HEENT: Keratoconjunctivitis sicca (dry inflammation of conjunctiva), malar rash (erythematous rash in "butterfly" pattern on the face), oral ulcers. Episcleritis or scleritis, xerophthalmia (dry eyes), parotid enlargement.

Chest: Pleural friction rub (pleuritis), fine rales (interstitial fibrosis).

Heart: Cardiac friction rubs (pericarditis).

Abdomen: Hepatosplenomegaly, abdominal tenderness.

Extremities: Joint tenderness, muscle weakness, lymphadenopathy sclerodactyly (thickening of digital subcutaneous tissue).

Labs: Electrolytes, creatinine, ANA, anti-Smith antibody, anti-DNA antibody, antineutrophilic cytoplasmic antibody, LE cell prep, RPR, ESR, CBC, UA, ECG, complement. UA (proteinuria, casts).

Diagnostic Criteria for Rheumatoid Arthritis: Four or more of the following.

1. Morning stiffness (>6 weeks)
2. Arthritis in 3 or more joints (>6 weeks)
3. Arthritis of hand joints (>6 weeks)
4. Symmetric arthritis (>6 weeks)
5. Rheumatoid nodules
6. Positive rheumatoid factor
7. X-ray abnormalities: Erosions, bony decalcification (especially in hands/wrist).

Diagnostic Criteria for Systemic Lupus Erythematosus: Four or more of the following.

1. Malar rash
2. Discoid rash
3. Photosensitivity

4. Oral or nasopharyngeal ulcers
5. Nonerosive arthritis
6. Pleuritis or pericarditis
7. Persistent proteinuria
8. Seizures or psychosis
9. Hemolytic anemia
10. Positive lupus erythematosus cell, positive anti-DNA antibody, Smith antibody, false positive VDRL.
11. Positive ANA

Psychiatric Disorders

Clinical Evaluation of the Psychiatric Patient

I. Psychiatric History

A. Identifying Information: Age, sex, marital status, race.

B. Chief Complaint (CC): Reason for consultation; often a direct quote from the patient.

C. History of Present Illness (HPI)

1. **Current Symptoms:** Date of onset, duration and course
2. Previous psychiatric symptoms and treatment
3. **Recent Psychosocial Stressors:** Stressful life events that may have contributed to the patient's current presentation
4. Reason the patient is presenting now
5. This section should provide evidence that supports or rules out the diagnosis.
6. **Suicidal Ideation.** Intent and planning.

D. Past Psychiatric History

1. Previous and current psychiatric diagnoses
2. History of psychiatric treatment, including outpatient and inpatient treatment
3. History of psychotropic medication use
4. History of suicide attempts

E. Past Medical History

1. Current and previous medical problems
2. Treatments, including prescription, over the counter medications, home or folk remedies.

F. Family History: Relatives with history of psychiatric disorders, suicide or suicide attempts, alcohol or substance abuse.

G. Social History

1. Source of income
2. Level of education, relationship history, including marriages and sexual orientation, number of children; individuals that currently live with patient.
3. Support network
4. Current alcohol or illicit drug usage
5. Occupational history

H. Developmental History: Family structure during childhood, relationships with parental figures and siblings; developmental milestones; peer relationships; school performance

II. **Mental Status Examination**
   A. **General Appearance and Behavior**
      1. Grooming, level of hygiene, characteristics of clothing
      2. Unusual physical characteristics or movements
      3. Attitude: Ability to interact with the interviewer
      4. Psychomotor activity: Agitation or psychomotor retardation
      5. Degree of eye contact
   B. **Affect**
      1. **Definition:** External range of expression observed by interviewer, described in terms of quality, range, and appropriateness
      2. **Types of Affect**
         a. Flat: Absence of all or most affect
         b. Blunted or restricted: Moderately reduced range of affect
         c. Labile: Intense changes in affect
         d. Full or wide range of affect: Appropriate affect
   C. **Mood:** Internal emotional tone of the patient (ie, dysphoric, euphoric, angry, euthymic, anxious).
   D. **Thought Processes**
      1. Use of Language: Quality and quantity of speech
      2. Rate, tone, associations and fluency of speech
   E. **Thought Content**
      1. **Definition:** Hallucinations, delusions and other perceptual disturbances
      2. **Thought Content Disorders**
         a. **Hallucinations:** False sensory perceptions; may be auditory, visual, tactile, gustatory or olfactory in nature.
         b. **Delusions:** Fixed, false beliefs, firmly held in spite of contradictory evidence.
         c. **Illusions:** Misinterpretations of reality
         d. **Derealization:** Feelings of unrealness involving the outer environment
   F. **Cognitive Evaluation**
      1. Level of consciousness
      2. **Orientation:** Person, place and date
      3. **Attention and Concentration:** Repeat 5 digits forwards and backwards or spell a five letter word ("world") forwards and backwards
      4. **Short-Term Memory:** Ability to recall 3 objects after 5 minutes
      5. **Fund of Knowledge:** Ability to name past five presidents or historical dates
      6. **Calculations:** Subtraction of serial 7s, simple math problems
      7. **Abstraction:** Proverb interpretation and similarities
   G. **Insight:** Does the patient display an understanding of his current problems? Does the patient understand the implication of these problems?

   H. **Judgment**
      1. Ability to make sound decisions regarding everyday activities
      2. Best evaluated by assessing a patient's history of decision making.
III. **DSM-IV Multiaxial Assessment Diagnosis**
   Axis I: Clinical Disorders
              Other conditions that may be a focus of clinical attention
   Axis II: Personality Disorders
              Mental Retardation
   Axis III: General Medical Conditions
   Axis IV: Psychosocial and Environmental Problems
   Axis V: Global Assessment of Functioning

Mini-mental Status Examination

Orientation: What is the year, season, day of week, date, month? - 5 points
  What is the state, county, city, hospital, floor ? - 5 points
Registration: Repeat: 3 objects: apple, book, coat. - 3 points
Attention/Calculation: Spell "WORLD" backwards - 5 points
Memory: Recall the names of the previous 3 objects: - 3 points
Language: Name a pencil and a watch - 2 points
  Repeat, "No ifs, and's or buts" - 1 point
  Three stage command: "Take this paper in your right hand, fold it in half, and
    put it on the floor." - 3 points
  Written command: "Close your eyes." - 1 point
  Write a sentence. - 1 point
Visual Spacial: Copy two overlapping pentagons - 1 point
Total Score
  Normal: 25-30
  Mild intellectual impairment: 20-25
  Moderate intellectual impairment: 10-20
  Severe intellectual impairment: 0-10

Attempted Suicide and Drug Overdose

History of the Present Illness: Time suicide was attempted and method.
  Quantity of pills; motive for attempt. Alcohol intake, other medications; place
  where medication was obtained; last menstrual period.
Symptoms of Tricyclic Antidepressant Overdose: Dry mouth, hallucinations,
  seizures, agitation, visual changes.
Psychiatric History: Previous suicide attempts or threats, family support,
  marital conflict, alcohol or drug abuse, sources of emotional stress.

Availability of other dangerous medications or weapons.

Precipitating factor for suicide attempt (death, divorce, humiliating event, unemployment, medical illness); further desire to commit suicide; is there a definite plan? Was action impulsive or planned?

Detailed account of events 48-hours prior to suicide attempt and events after. Feelings of sadness, guilt, hopelessness, helplessness. Reasons that a patient has to wish to go on living. Did the patient believe that he would succeed in suicide? Is the patient upset that he is still alive?

Personal or family history of emotional, physical, or sexual abuse.

Family history of depression, suicide, psychiatric disease.

Physical Examination

General Appearance: Level of consciousness, confusion, delirium; presence of potentially dangerous objects or substances (belts, shoe laces).

Vital Signs: BP (hypotension), pulse (bradycardia), temperature (hyperpyrexia), respiratory rate.

HEENT: Signs of trauma; pupil size and reactivity, mydriasis, nystagmus.

Chest: Abnormal respiratory patterns, rhonchi (aspiration).

Heart: Rhythm (arrhythmias).

Abdomen: Decreased bowel sounds.

Extremities: Needle marks, wounds, ecchymoses.

Neuro: Mental status exam; tremor, clonus, hyperactive reflexes.

ECG Signs of Antidepressant Overdose: QRS widening, PR or QT interval prolongation, AV block, ventricular tachycardia, Torsades de pointes vertricular arrhythmia.

Labs: Electrolytes, BUN, creatinine, glucose; ABG. Alcohol, acetaminophen levels; chest x-ray, urine toxicology screen.

Alcohol Withdrawal

History of the Present Illness: Determine the amount and frequency of alcohol use and other drug use in the past month, week, and day. Time of last alcohol consumption; tremors, anxiety, nausea, vomiting; diaphoresis, agitation, fever, abdominal pain, headaches; hematemesis, melena, past withdrawal reactions; history of delirium tremens, hallucinations, chest pain.

Determine whether the patient ever consumes five or more drinks at a time (binge drinking). Previous abuse of alcohol or other drugs.

Effects of the alcohol or drug use on the patient's life may include problems with health, family, job or financial status or with the legal system.

History of blackouts or motor vehicle crashes; affect of alcohol use on family members.

Past Medical History: Gastritis, ulcers, GI bleeding; hepatitis, cirrhosis, pancreatitis, drug abuse. Age of onset of heavy drinking.

Family history of alcoholism.

Physical Examination

General Appearance: Poor nutritional status, slurred speech, disorientation, diaphoresis.

Vital Signs: BP (hypertension), pulse (tachycardia), respiratory rate, temperature (hyper/hypothermia).

HEENT: Signs of head trauma, ecchymoses. Conjunctival injection, icterus, nystagmus, extraocular movements, pupil reactivity.

Chest: Rhonchi, crackles (aspiration), gynecomastia (cirrhosis).

Heart: Rate and rhythm, murmurs.

Abdomen: Liver tenderness, hepatomegaly or liver atrophy, liver span, splenomegaly, ascites.

Genitourinary: Testicular atrophy, hernias.

Rectal: Occult blood.

Skin: Jaundice, spider angiomas (stellate arterioles with branching capillaries), palmar erythema, muscle atrophy (stigmata of liver disease); needle tracks.

Neuro: Cranial nerves 2-12, reflexes, ataxia. Asterixis, decreased vibratory sense (peripheral neuropathy).

Wernicke's Encephalopathy: Ophthalmoplegia, ataxia, confusion (thiamine deficiency).

Korsakoff's Syndrome: Retrograde or antegrade amnesia, confabulation.

Labs: Electrolytes, magnesium, glucose, CBC, liver function tests, UA; chest X-ray; ECG.

Differential Diagnosis of Altered Mental Status: Alcohol intoxication, hypoglycemia, narcotic overdose, meningitis, drug overdose, head trauma, alcoholic ketoacidosis, anticholinergic poisoning, sedative-hypnotic withdrawal, intracranial hemorrhage.

Commonly Used Formulas

A-a gradient = $[(P_B - PH_2O) FiO_2 - PCO_2/R] - PO_2$ arterial

= $(713 \times FiO2 - pCO2/0.8) - pO2$ arterial

P_B = 760 mmHg; PH_2O = 47 mmHg; R ≈ 0.8
normal Aa gradient <10-15 mmHg (room air)

Arterial oxygen capacity = (Hgb(gm)/100 mL) x 1.36 mL O2/gm Hgb

Arterial O2 content = 1.36(Hgb)(SaO2)+0.003(PaO2)= NL 20 vol%

O2 delivery = CO x arterial O2 content = NL 640-1000 mL O2/min

Cardiac output = HR x stroke volume

$$CO\ L/min = \frac{125\ mL\ O2/min/M^2}{8.5\ \{(1.36)(Hgb)(SaO2) - (1.36)(Hgb)(SvO2)\}} \times 100$$

Normal CO = 4-6 L/min

$$SVR = \frac{MAP - CVP \times 80}{CO_{L/min}} = NL\ 800\text{-}1200\ dyne/sec/cm^2$$

$$PVR = \frac{PA - PCWP \times 80}{CO_{L/min}} = NL\ 45\text{-}120\ dyne/sec/cm^2$$

$$GFR\ mL/min = \frac{(140 - age) \times wt\ in\ Kg}{\substack{72\ (males) \times serum\ Cr\ (mg/dL) \\ 85\ (females) \times serum\ Cr\ (mg/dL)}}$$

$$Creatinine\ clearance = \frac{U\ Cr\ (mg/100\ mL) \times U\ vol\ (mL)}{P\ Cr\ (mg/100\ mL) \times time\ (1440\ min\ for\ 24h)}$$

Normal creatinine clearance = 100-125 mL/min(males), 85-105(females)

$$Body\ water\ deficit\ (L) = \frac{0.6(weight\ kg)([measured\ serum\ Na]-140)}{140}$$

$$Osmolality\ mOsm/kg = 2[Na+ K] + \frac{BUN}{2.8} + \frac{glucose}{18} = NL\ 270\text{-}290\ \frac{mOsm}{kg}$$

$$Fractional\ excreted\ Na = \frac{U\ Na/\ Serum\ Na \times 100}{U\ Cr/\ Serum\ Cr} = NL<1\%$$

Anion Gap = Na - (Cl + HCO3)

For each 100 mg/dL increase in glucose, Na+ decrease by 1.6 mEq/L.

Corrected serum Ca+ (mg/dL) = measured Ca mg/dL + 0.8 x (4 - albumin g/dL)

Ideal body weight males = 50 kg for first 5 feet of height + 2.3 kg for each additional inch.

Ideal body weight females = 45.5 kg for first 5 feet + 2.3 kg for each additional inch.

Basal energy expenditure (BEE):
Males=66 + (13.7 x actual weight Kg) + (5 x height cm)-(6.8 x age)
Females= 655+(9.6 x actual weight Kg)+(1.7 x height cm)-(4.7 x age)

Nitrogen Balance = Gm protein intake/6.25 - urine urea nitrogen - (3-4 gm/d insensible loss)

Predicted Maximal Heart Rate = 220 - age

Normal ECG Intervals (sec)

PR	0.12-0.20
QRS	0.06-0.08
Heart rate/min	**Q-T**
60	0.33-0.43
70	0.31-0.41
80	0.29-0.38
90	0.28-0.36
100	0.27-0.35

Commonly Used Drug Levels

Drug	Therapeutic Range
Amikacin	Peak 25-30; trough <10 mcg/mL
Amitriptyline	100-250 ng/mL
Carbamazepine	4-10 mcg/mL
Desipramine	150-300 ng/mL
Digoxin	0.8-2.0 ng/mL
Disopyramide	2-5 mcg/mL
Doxepin	75-200 ng/mL
Flecainide	0.2-1.0 mcg/mL
Gentamicin	Peak 6.0-8.0; trough <2.0 mcg/mL
Imipramine	150-300 ng/mL
Lidocaine	2-5 mcg/mL
Lithium	0.5-1.4 mEq/L
Nortriptyline	50-150 ng/mL
Phenobarbital	10-30 mEq/mL
Phenytoin	8-20 mcg/mL
Procainamide	4.0-8.0 mcg/mL
Quinidine	2.5-5.0 mcg/mL
Salicylate	15-25 mg/dL
Streptomycin	Peak 10-20; trough <5 mcg/mL
Theophylline	8-20 mcg/mL
Tocainide	4-10 mcg/mL
Valproic acid	50-100 mcg/mL
Vancomycin	Peak 30-40; trough <10 mcg/mL

Commonly Used Abbreviations

1/2 NS	0.45% saline solution	CO₂	carbon dioxide
ac	ante cibum (before meals)	COPD	chronic obstructive pulmonary disease
ABG	arterial blood gas	CPK-MB	myocardial-specific CPK isoenzyme
ac	before meals		
ACTH	adrenocorticotropic hormone	CPR	cardiopulmonary resuscitation
ad lib	ad libitum (as needed or desired)	CSF	cerebrospinal fluid
		CT	computerized tomography
ADH	antidiuretic hormone	CVP	central venous pressure
AFB	acid-fast bacillus	CXR	chest x-ray
alk phos	alkaline phosphatase	d/c	discharge; discontinue
		D5W	5% dextrose water solution; also D10W, D50W
ALT	alanine aminotransferase	DIC	disseminated intravascular coagulation
am	morning	diff	differential count
AMA	against medical advice	DKA	diabetic ketoacidosis
		dL	deciliter
amp	ampule	DOSS	docusate sodium sulfosuccinate
AMV	assisted mandatory ventilation; assist mode ventilation		
		DT's	delirium tremens
ANA	antinuclear antibody	ECG	electrocardiogram
ante	before	ER	emergency room
AP	anteroposterior	ERCP	endoscopic retrograde cholangiopancreatography
ARDS	adult respiratory distress syndrome		
		ESR	erythrocyte sedimentation rate
ASA	acetylsalicylic acid	ET	endotracheal tube
AST	aspartate aminotransferase	ETOH	alcohol
		Fe/TIBC	iron/total iron-binding capacity
bid	bis in die (twice a day)	Fe	iron
B-12	vitamin B-12 (cyanocobalamin)	FEV₁	forced expiratory volume (in one second)
BM	bowel movement	FiO2	fractional inspired oxygen
BP	blood pressure	g	gram(s)
BUN	blood urea nitrogen	GC	gonococcal; gonococcus
c/o	complaint of	GFR	glomerular filtration rate
c̄	cum (with)	GI	gastrointestinal
C and S	culture and sensitivity	gm	gram
		gt	drop
C	centigrade	gtt	drops
Ca	calcium	h	hour
cap	capsule	H20	water
CBC	complete blood count; includes hemoglobin, hematocrit, red blood cell indices, white blood cell count, and platelets	HBsAG	hepatitis B surface antigen
		HCO3	bicarbonate
		Hct	hematocrit
		HDL	high-density lipoprotein
		Hg	mercury
		Hgb	hemoglobin concentration
		HIV	human immunodeficiency virus
cc	cubic centimeter		
CCU	coronary care unit	hr	hour
cm	centimeter	hs	hora somni (bedtime, hour of sleep)
CMF	cyclophosphamide, methotrexate, fluorouracil		
		IM	intramuscular
CNS	central nervous system	I and O	intake and output--measurement of the patient's intake and output, including urine,

	vomit, diarrhea, and drainage
IU	international units
ICU	intensive care unit
IgM	immunoglobulin M
IMV	intermittent mandatory ventilation
INH	isoniazid
INR	International normalized ratio
IPPB	intermittent positive-pressure breathing
IV	intravenous or intravenously
IVP	intravenous pyelogram; intravenous piggyback
K^+	potassium
kcal	kilocalorie
KCL	potassium chloride
KPO4	potassium phosphate
KUB	x-ray of abdomen (kidneys, ureters, bowels)
L	liter
LDH	lactate dehydrogenase
LDL	low-density lipoprotein
liq	liquid
LLQ	left lower quadrant
LP	lumbar puncture, low potency
LR	lactated Ringer's (solution)
MB	myocardial band
MBC	minimal bacterial concentration
mcg	microgram
mEq	milliequivalent
mg	milligram
Mg	magnesium
MgSO4	Magnesium Sulfate
MI	myocardial infarction
MIC	minimum inhibitory concentration
mL	milliliter
mm	millimeter
MOM	Milk of Magnesia
MRI	magnetic resonance imaging
Na	sodium
NaHCO3	sodium bicarbonate
Neuro	neurologic
NG	nasogastric
NKA	no known allergies
NPH	neutral protamine Hagedorn (insulin)
NPO	nulla per os (nothing by mouth)
NS	normal saline solution (0.9%)
NSAID	nonsteroidal anti-inflammatory drug
O2	oxygen
OD	right eye
oint	ointment
OS	left eye
Osm	osmolality
OT	occupational therapy
OTC	over the counter
OU	each eye
oz	ounce
p, post	after
pc	post cibum (after meals)
PA	posteroanterior; pulmonary artery
PaO2	arterial oxygen pressure
pAO2	partial pressure of oxygen in alveolar gas
PB	phenobarbital
pc	after meals
pCO2	partial pressure of carbon dioxide
PEEP	positive end-expiratory pressure
per	by
pH	hydrogen ion concentration (H+)
PID	pelvic inflammatory disease
pm	afternoon
PO	orally, per os
pO2	partial pressure of oxygen
polys	polymorphonuclear leukocytes
PPD	purified protein derivative
PR	per rectum
prn	pro re nata (as needed)
PT	physical therapy; prothrombin time
PTCA	percutaneous transluminal coronary angioplasty
PTT	partial thromboplastin time
PVC	premature ventricular contraction
q	quaque (every) q6h, q2h every 6 hours; every 2 hours
qid	quarter in die (four times a day)
qAM	every morning
qd	quaque die (every day)
qh	every hour
qhs	every night before bedtime
qid	4 times a day
qOD	every other day
qs	quantity sufficient
R/O	rule out
RA	rheumatoid arthritis; room air; right atrial
Resp	respiratory rate
RL	Ringer's lactated solution (also LR)
ROM	range of motion
rt	right
s	sine (without)

s/p	status post (the condition of being after)	URI	upper respiratory infection
sat	saturated	Ut Dict	as directed
SBP	systolic blood pressure	UTI	urinary tract infection
		VAC	vincristine, adriamycin, and cyclophosphamide
SC	subcutaneously	vag	vaginal
SIADH	syndrome of inappropriate antidiuretic hormone	VC	vital capacity
		VDRL	Venereal Disease Research Laboratory
SL	sublingually under tongue	VF	ventricular function
		V fib	ventricular fibrillation
SLE	systemic lupus erythematosus	VLDL	very low-density lipoprotein
SMA-12	sequential multiple analysis; a panel of 12 chemistry tests. Tests include Na$^+$, K$^+$, HCO3 , Chloride , BUN, glucose, creatinine, bilirubin, calcium, total protein, albumin, and alkaline phosphatase. Other chemistry panels include SMA-6 and SMA-20	Vol	volume
		VS	vital signs
		VT	ventricular tachycardia
		W	water
		WBC	white blood count
		x	times
SMX	sulfamethoxazole		
sob	shortness of breath		
sol	solution		
SQ	under the skin		
ss	one-half		
STAT	statim (immediately)		
susp	suspension		
tid	ter in die (three times a day)		
T4	Thyroxine level (T4)		
T3RU	Triiodothyronine resin uptake		
tab	tablet		
TB	tuberculosis		
Tbsp	tablespoon		
Temp	temperature		
TIA	transient ischemic attack		
tid	three times a day		
TKO	to keep open, an infusion rate (500 mL/24h) just enough to keep the IV from clotting		
TMP	trimethoprim		
TMP-SMX	trimethoprim-sulfamethoxazole combination		
TPA	tissue plasminogen activator		
TSH	thyroid-stimulating hormone		
tsp	teaspoon		
U	units		
UA	urinalysis		
ung	ointment		

Index